McMinn's
Color Atlas of

Foot and Ankle Anatomy

Commissioning Editors: Richard Furn and Inta Ozols
Project Development Manager: Duncan Fraser
Project Manager: Jess Thompson
Illustration Manager: Bruce Hogarth
Designer: George Ajayi
Page Layout: Jim Hope (PTU Elsevier)

THIRD EDITION

McMinn's
Color Atlas of
Foot and Ankle Anatomy

Bari M. Logan MA, FMA, Hon MBIE, MAMAA

University Prosector
Department of Anatomy
University of Cambridge
Cambridge, UK

Dishan Singh MBChB, FRCS(Orth)

Consultant Orthopaedic Surgeon
Foot and Ankle Unit
Royal National Orthopaedic Hospital
Stanmore, UK

Ralph T. Hutchings

Photographer for Imagingbody.com
Formerly Chief Medical Laboratory Scientific Officer
Royal College of Surgeons of England
London, UK

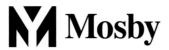

EDINBURGH LONDON NEW YORK OXFORD PHILADELPHIA ST LOUIS SYDNEY TORONTO 2004

MOSBY
An imprint of Elsevier Limited

First edition 1982
Second edition 1996
Third edition 2004

ISBN 0723431930

British Library Cataloguing in Publication Data
A catalogue record for this book is available from the British Library

Library of Congress Cataloging in Publication Data
A catalog record for this book is available from the Library of Congress

Notice
Medical knowledge is constantly changing. Standard safety precautions must be followed, but as new research and clinical experience broaden our knowledge, changes in treatment and drug therapy may become necessary or appropriate. Readers are advised to check the most current product information provided by the manufacturer of each drug to be administered to verify the recommended dose, the method and duration of administration, and contraindications. It is the responsibility of the practitioner, relying on experience and knowledge of the patient, to determine dosages and the best treatment for each individual patient. Neither the Publisher nor the authors assume any liability for any injury and/or damage to persons or property arising from this publication.
The Publisher

The
publisher's
policy is to use
**paper manufactured
from sustainable forests**

Printed in Spain

Last digit is the print number : 9 8 7 6 5 4 3 2 1

Contents

Imaging of the Foot and Ankle

4

Appendices

Preface

This book was first penned by the hand of Professor R. M. H. McMinn in 1981 in response to the suggestion from the publisher Peter Wolfe, "for a specific anatomical text to suit the educational requirements of chiropodists and podiatrists in training".
It has proved a very popular book and this third edition heralds twenty-one years of publication in six language editions of English, Japanese, French, German, Dutch and Spanish.

With the full retirement of 'Bob' McMinn to the Scottish Highlands, a new author, Dishan Singh, joins the team and as a specialist clinician he brings a new level of expertise to the books content.
In order to meet readers demands, the two main features that we have included are new prosections relating to the structure of the male and female pelvis and four pages of magnetic resonance images of the foot and ankle region. We hope that these new additions will be appreciated and that the book will continue in its popularity.

Although the book now truly extends to cover the whole of the lower limb, by tradition we retain the title 'Foot and Ankle Anatomy', and incorporate 'McMinn' as a tribute to our distinguished colleague and outstanding anatomist.

New terminology

The Greek adjective 'peroneal' (see page 45) is now replaced by the Latin 'fibular' for various muscles, vessels, nerves and structures. For example: Fibularis tertius instead of Peroneal tertius; Fibular artery instead of Peroneal artery; Common fibular nerve instead of Common peroneal nerve; Inferior fibular retinaculum instead of Inferior peroneal retinaculum.
For this new edition, in order to ease in the new terminology for those used to working from older texts, the term peroneal is included italicised in brackets; e.g. Deep fibular (*peroneal*) nerve.

Also note, flexor accessorius is now known as quadratus plantae.

This terminology conforms to the International Anatomical Terminology — Terminologia Anatomica — created in 1988 by the Federative Committee on Anatomical Terminology (FCAT) and approved by the 56 Member Associations of the International Federation of Associations of Anatomists (IFAA).

Acknowledgements

The authors are indebted to the following:

- Dr Ian G. Parkin, Clinical Anatomist, University of Cambridge, for expert anatomical knowledge.
- Mr Martin Watson, Mel Lazenby and Lucie Whitehead, Department of Anatomy, University of Cambridge, for preservation of anatomical material.
- Mr Adrian Newman, Mr Ian Bolton and Mr John Bashford, Audio Visual Unit, Department of Anatomy, University of Cambridge, for photographic expertise and advice.
- Dr Peter Baxter, Mr John Bridger, Dr Brendan Burchell, Dr Simon Poole and Mr Robert Whitaker, of Cambridge, for much appreciated support and guidance.
- Inta Ozols, Duncan Fraser, Jessica Thompson, and all the team at Elsevier for their help, advice and support during the preparation of this book.

Radiographs
- Dr Peter Abrahams p. 96 D and E
- Dr Oscar Craig p. 21 B
- Dr Kate Stevens p. 29 C, p.108 B, p. 110 A and B
- Mr W Stripp p.111 C and D

MRIs
- Dr Paul O'Donnell pp. 112–115

Dedications

To Robert Logan
    – Bari M. Logan

To Prema, my wife
    – Dishan Singh

In memory of Peter Wolfe
    – Ralph T. Hutchings

Orientation

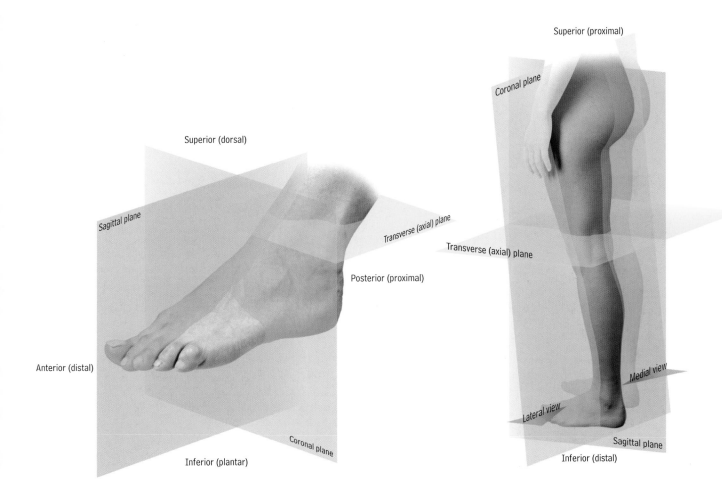

Superior (dorsal)

Sagittal plane

Transverse (axial) plane

Posterior (proximal)

Anterior (distal)

Coronal plane

Inferior (plantar)

Superior (proximal)

Coronal plane

Transverse (axial) plane

Medial view

Lateral view

Sagittal plane

Inferior (distal)

Lower Limb, Pelvis and Hip

1

Lower limb survey
Bones, muscles and surface landmarks of the left lower limb, from the front

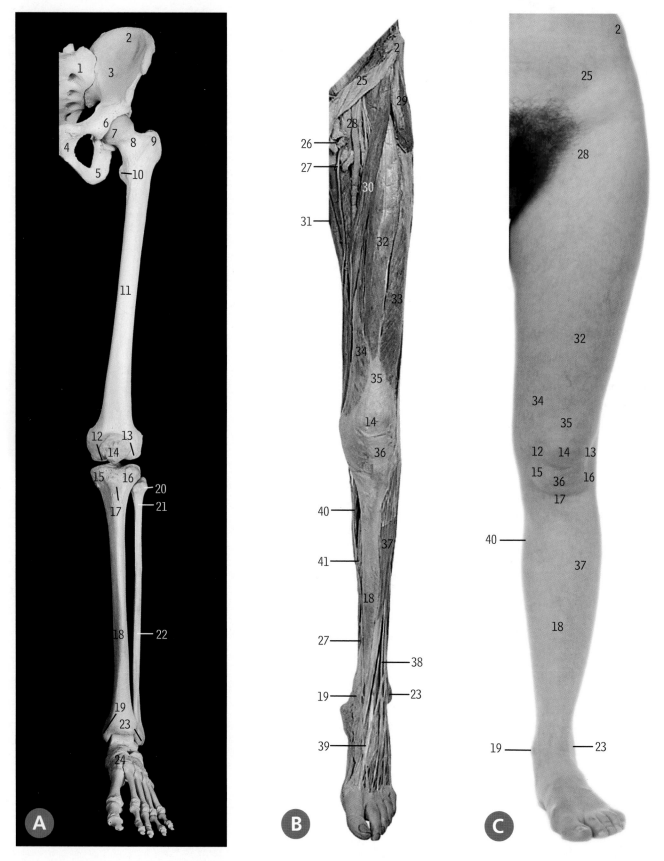

1 Sacrum
2 Iliac crest
3 Ilium ⎫
4 Pubis ⎬ of hip bone
5 Ischium ⎭
6 Rim of acetabulum
7 Head ⎫
8 Neck │
9 Greater trochanter │
10 Lesser trochanter ⎬ of femur
11 Body (shaft) │
12 Medial condyle │
13 Lateral condyle ⎭
14 Patella
15 Medial condyle ⎫
16 Lateral condyle │
17 Tuberosity ⎬ of tibia
18 Body (shaft) │
19 Medial malleolus ⎭
20 Head ⎫
21 Neck ⎬ of fibula
22 Body (shaft) │
23 Lateral malleolus ⎭
24 Foot
25 Inguinal ligament
26 Inguinal lymph nodes
27 Great saphenous vein
28 Femoral triangle, vessels and nerve
29 Tensor fasciae latae
30 Sartorius
31 Gracilis
32 Rectus femoris
33 Vastus lateralis
34 Vastus medialis
35 Quadriceps tendon
36 Patellar ligament
37 Tibialis anterior
38 Extensor digitorum longus
39 Extensor hallucis longus
40 Gastrocnemius
41 Soleus

Ⓐ Bones of the left lower limb, from the front

Ⓑ Muscles of the left lower limb, from the front

Ⓒ Surface landmarks of the left lower limb, from the front

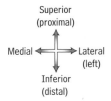

- The main parts or regions of the lower limb are the gluteal region (consisting of the hip at the side and the buttock at the back), the thigh, the knee, the leg, the ankle and the foot. The term *leg* properly refers to the part between the knee and the foot, although it is commonly used for the whole lower limb.

- The hip bone consists of three bones fused together—the ilium (**3**), ischium (**5**) and pubis (**4**) — and forms a pelvic girdle. The two hip bones or girdles unite with each other in front at the pubic symphysis (p. 18, **B33**), and at the back they join the sacrum at the sacro-iliac joints (p. 18, **A7** and **C6**), so forming the bony pelvis.

- The femur (**11**) is the bone of the thigh; the tibia (**18**) and fibula (**22**) are the bones of the leg.

- The acetabulum (**6**) of the hip bone and the head of the femur (**7**) form the hip joint (p. 18, **A12** and **14**, **B18** and **20**, **C18** and **20**).

- The condyles of the femur (**12** and **13**) and tibia (**15** and **16**) together with the patella (**14**) form the knee joint.

- The head of the fibula (**20**) forms a small joint with the tibia, the superior tibiofibular joint. The inferior tibiofibular joint, properly called the tibiofibular syndesmosis (a type of fibrous joint), is a fibrous union between the tibia and fibula just above the ankle joint.

- The ankle is the lower part of the leg in the region of the ankle joint (p. 54, 56, 58 and 60).

- The lower ends of the tibia (**18**) and fibula (**22**) articulate with the talus of the foot to form the ankle joint (p. 54 and 56).

- The body of a long bone is commonly called the shaft.

- The adjective 'peroneal' (Greek, see p. 43) is now replaced by the Latin 'fibular' for various vessels and nerves, e.g., common fibular nerve instead of common peroneal nerve. See notes on New Terminology p. vii.

For details of limb muscles, nerves and arteries see the Appendix:

Muscles—pp. 115–119, including **Figs. 2–7**.

Nerves—pp. 120–122, including **Figs. 8–11**.

Arteries—pp. 123 and 124, including **Figs. 12** and **13**.

Lower limb survey
Bones, muscles and surface landmarks of the left lower limb, from behind

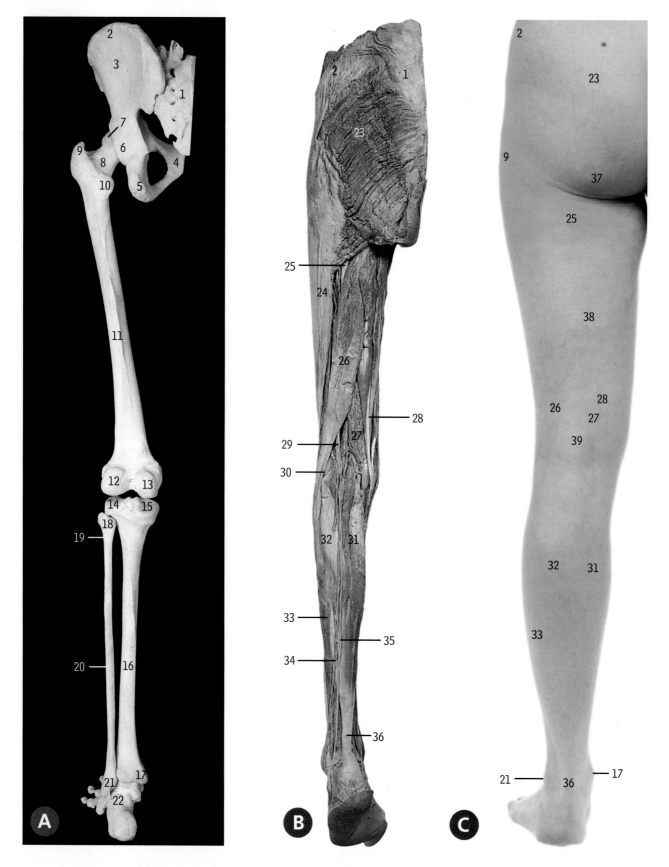

1 Sacrum
2 Iliac crest
3 Ilium
4 Pubis
5 Ischium
6 Rim of acetabulum
7 Head ⎤
8 Neck │
9 Greater trochanter │ of femur
10 Lesser trochanter │
11 Body │
12 Lateral condyle │
13 Medial conyle ⎦
14 Lateral condyle ⎤
15 Medial condyle │ of tibia
16 Body │
17 Medial malleolus ⎦
18 Head ⎤
19 Neck │ of fibula
20 Body │
21 Lateral malleolus ⎦
22 Foot
23 Gluteus maximus
24 Iliotibial tract
25 Sciatic nerve
26 Biceps femoris
27 Semimembranosus
28 Semitendinosus
29 Tibial nerve
30 Common fibular (*peroneal*) nerve
31 Medial head ⎤ of gastrocnemius
32 Lateral head ⎦
33 Soleus
34 Sural nerve
35 Small saphenous vein
36 Tendo calcaneus
37 Fold of buttock (gluteal fold)
38 Hamstring muscles
39 Popliteal fossa

- The curved fold of the buttock (**37**) does not correspond to the straight (but oblique) lower border of gluteus maximus (**23**).

- The tendons of gastrocnemius (**31** and **32**) and soleus (**33**) join to form the tendo calcaneus (**36**), known commonly as the Achilles' tendon.

- The muscles on the back of the thigh with prominent tendons—semimembranosus (**27**), semitendinosus (**28**) and biceps femoris (long head, **26**)—are known commonly as the hamstrings (see the note on p. 27).

A Bones of the left lower, limb from behind

B Muscles of the left lower limb, from behind

C Surface landmarks of the left lower limb, from behind

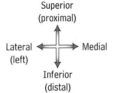

Superior
(proximal)

Lateral ⟷ Medial
(left)

Inferior
(distal)

Lower limb survey
Bones, muscles and surface landmarks of the left lower limb, from the medial side

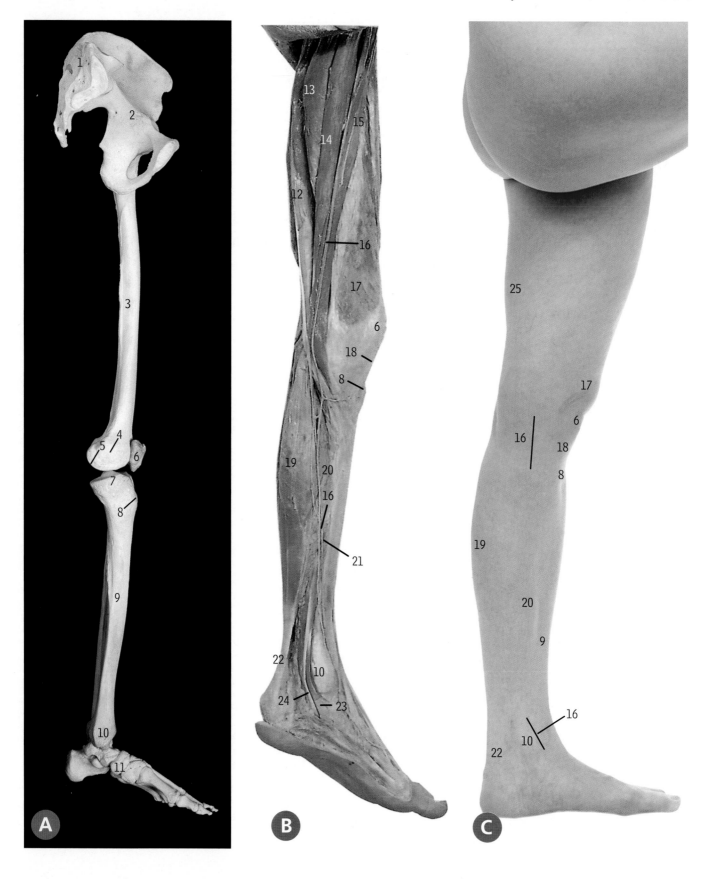

1 Sacrum
2 Hip bone
3 Body ⎫
4 Medial epicondyle ⎬ of femur
5 Medial condyle ⎭
6 Patella
7 Medial condyle ⎫
8 Tuberosity ⎪
9 Body ⎬ of tibia
10 Medial malleolus ⎭
11 Foot
12 Semitendinosus
13 Semimembranosus
14 Gracilis
15 Sartorius
16 Great saphenous vein
17 Vastus medialis
18 Patellar ligament
19 Gastrocnemius
20 Soleus
21 Saphenous nerve
22 Tendo calcaneus
23 Tibialis posterior
24 Flexor digitorum longus
25 Hamstrings

• At the ankle the great saphenous vein (**16**), the longest vein in the body, passes upwards in front of the medial malleolus (**10**). At the knee it lies a hand's breadth behind the medial border of the patella (**6**). It ends by draining into the femoral vein (p. 24, **12** and **18**).

A Bones of the left lower limb, from the medial side

B Muscles of the left lower limb, from the medial side

C Surface landmarks of the left lower limb, from the medial side

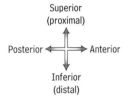

Superior
(proximal)

Posterior ←——→ Anterior

Inferior
(distal)

Lower limb survey
Bones, muscles and surface landmarks of the left lower limb, from the lateral side

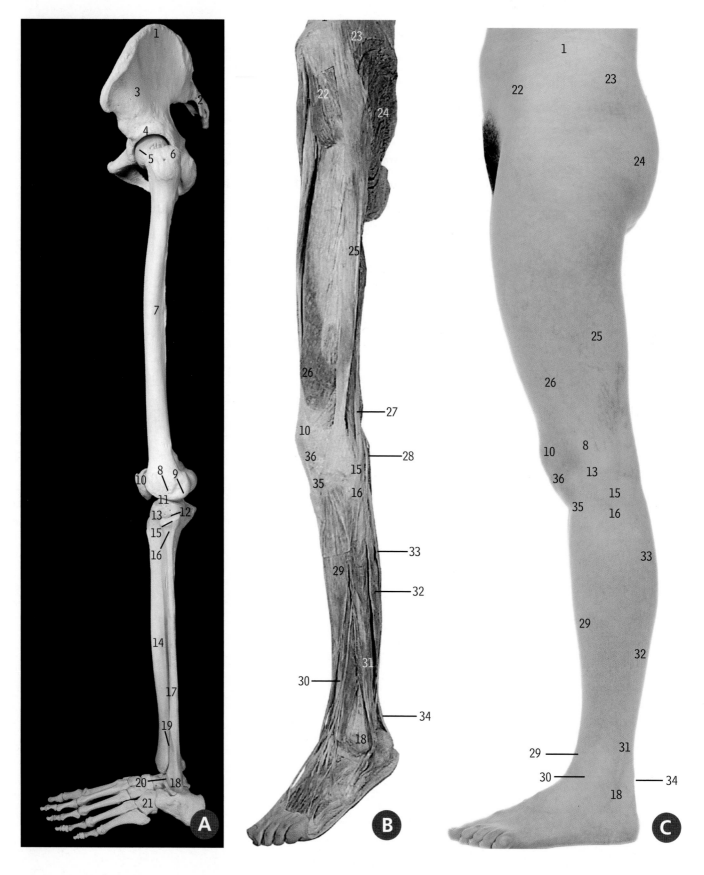

1 Iliac crest
2 Sacrum
3 Hip bone
4 Hip joint
5 Head
6 Greater trochanter
7 Body } of femur
8 Lateral epicondyle
9 Lateral condyle
10 Patella
11 Knee joint
12 Superior tibiofibular joint
13 Lateral condyle } of tibia
14 Body
15 Head
16 Neck } of fibula
17 Body
18 Lateral malleolus
19 Inferior tibiofibular joint
20 Ankle joint
21 Foot
22 Tensor fasciae latae
23 Gluteus medius
24 Gluteus maximus
25 Iliotibial tract
26 Vastus lateralis
27 Biceps femoris
28 Common fibular (peroneal) nerve
29 Tibialis anterior
30 Extensor digitorum longus
31 Fibularis (peroneus) longus
32 Soleus
33 Gastrocnemius
34 Tendo calcaneus
35 Tibial tuberosity
36 Patellar ligament

- The common fibular (*peroneal*) nerve (**28**), the only *palpable* major nerve of the lower limb, can be felt as it passes downward and forward across the neck of the fibula (**16**).

A Bones of the left lower limb, from the lateral side

B Muscles of the left lower limb, from the lateral side

C Surface landmarks of the left lower limb, from the lateral side

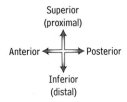
Superior
(proximal)

Anterior ← → Posterior

Inferior
(distal)

Male pelvic viscera and vessels

seen on the right side in a sagittal section, after removal of most of the peritoneum (serous membrane)

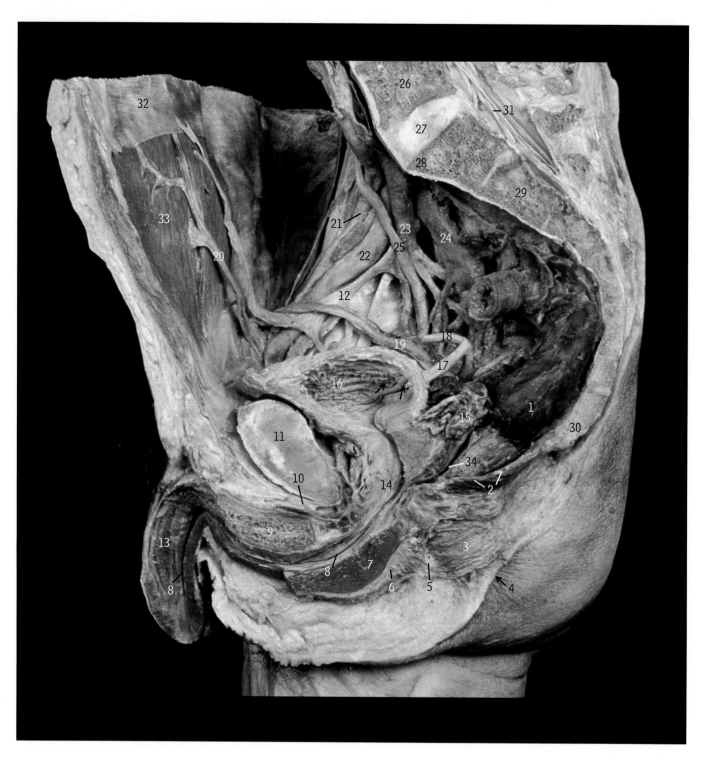

The section is mostly in the midline; small bowel, large bowel and peritoneum (serous membrane) have been removed but the whole of the anal canal and the lower part of the left levator ani muscle have been preserved to show the external anal sphincter (as in the female section, p. 12).

1 Rectum
2 Cut edge of levator ani
3 External anal sphincter covering anal canal
4 Anus, above arrowhead
5 Perineal body
6 Bulbospongiosus overlying corpus spongiosum
7 Corpus spongiosum, the part of the penis containing the urethra
8 Spongy part of urethra, within the corpus spongiosum
9 Corpus cavernosum of penis
10 Deep dorsal vein of penis, draining back to the vesicoprostatic venous plexus, the sponge-like tissue sectioned here in front of the prostate
11 Pubic symphysis
12 Superior vesical artery
13 Corpus cavernosum of penis
14 Prostate and prostatic part of urethra
15 Left seminal vesicle, cut in section
16 Bladder, with uretral openings marked with arrows
17 Left ureter
18 Left ductus (vas) deferens
19 Right ductus (vas) deferens
20 Inferior epigastric vessels
21 External iliac artery
22 External iliac vein
23 Internal iliac artery
24 Internal iliac vein
25 Ureter
26 Body of fifth lumbar vertebra
27 Fifth lumbar intervertebral disc
28 Promontory of sacrum
29 Sacrum
30 Coccyx
31 Cauda equina within sacral canal
32 Posterior wall of rectus sheath
33 Rectus abdominis
34 Rectovesical pouch

- The ureters (**17**, **25**) conduct urine from the kidneys to the bladder (**16**) where it is stored until sensation of volume dictates expulsion via the single tube of the urethra (**8**), the extent of its full length seen here laying within the bisected shaft of the penis (**7**).

- The single prostate gland (**14**) and the paired seminal vesicals (**15**, left) are accessory secretory sex glands which produce most of the volume of seminal fluid.

- The prostate gland (**14**), normally the size of a chestnut, lies just below the bladder (**16**) and opens into the urethra (**8**); The seminal vesicals (**15**, left) open into the ductus (vas) deferens (**18**, **19**) which conduct sperm from the epididymus of each testis to the urethra (**8**) on ejaculation.

- The rectum (**1**) is the terminal part of the large intestine (colon) where faeces collect prior to defecation via the anus (**4**) the opening and closing of which is controlled by the muscles which form the external sphincter (**3**). The space between the rectum (**1**), prostate gland (**14**) and seminal vesicals (**15**, left) is known as the retrovesicle pouch (**34**).

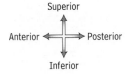

Female pelvic viscera and vessels *seen on the right side in a sagittal section, after removal of most of the peritoneum (serous membrane)*

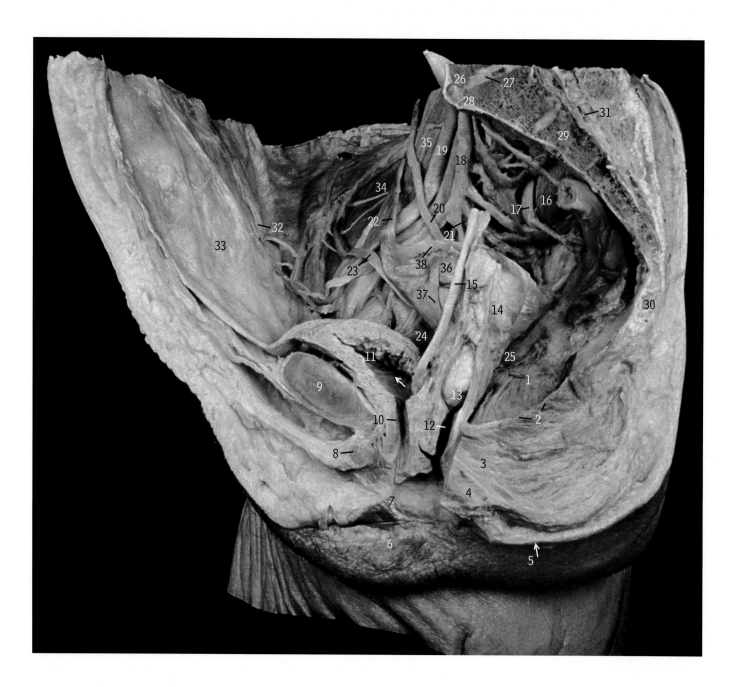

The section is mostly in the midline; small bowel, large bowel and much of the peritoneum (serous membrane) have been removed but the whole of the anal canal and the lower part of the left levator ani muscle have been preserved to show the external anal sphincter, (as in the male section, p. 10).

1 Rectum
2 Cut edge of left levator ani
3 External anal sphincter covering anal canal
4 Perineal body (central perineal tendon)
5 Anus, above arrowhead
6 Labium majus
7 Labium minus
8 Clitoris
9 Pubic symphysis
10 Urethra, surrounded by sphincter urethrae
11 Bladder, arrow points to right ureter
12 Vagina
13 Cervix of uterus
14 Body of uterus
15 Left ureter
16 Piriformis
17 Anterior ramus of S1 nerve
18 External iliac vein
19 External iliac artery

20 Right ureter
21 Internal iliac vessels and branches
22 Ovarian vessels
23 Round ligament of uterus
24 Vesico-uterine pouch
25 Recto-uterine pouch (of Douglas)
26 Body of fifth lumbar vertebra
27 Fifth lumbar intervertebral disc
28 Promontory of sacrum
29 Sacrum
30 Coccyx
31 Sacral canal
32 Inferior epigastric vessels
33 Peritoneum overlying rectus abdominis [see 32–33, p. 10]
34 Iliacus
35 Psoas major
36 Right ovary
37 Right uterine (fallopian tube)
38 Right broad ligament

- The vagina (12) is the lower part of the female reproductive tract and lies in a central position between, anteriorly the bladder (11) and posteriorly the rectum (1); Superiorly, it connects the lower end of the uterus (the cervix) (13) with inferiorly, the margin of the vaginal orifice and the labium majus (6) and labium minus (7).

- The urethra (10) in the female is much shorter in length, being only 4cm, compared to that in the male, usually 18cm; from the bladder it opens into the vaginal vestibule a few centimetres behind the clitoris (8). The space between the bladder (11) and the uterus (14) is known as the vesico-uterine pouch (24) and between the uterus (14) and the rectum (1) the recto-uterine pouch (of Douglas), (25).

- The body of the uterus (14) is pear shaped and normally lies over the bladder (11), from its sides the broad ligament (38, right) extends to the lateral walls of the pelvis, these help to keep the uterus in a central position.

- The ovaries (36, right) are suspended by part of the broad ligament (mesovarium) close to the lateral walls of the pelvis and are the main female reproductive organs, they produce cyclic steroid hormones as well as ovum (egg cells). The open ends of the uterine (fallopian) tubes (37, right) are positioned close to the ovaries thus enabelling discharged ova to freely enter them.

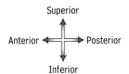

Gluteal region
Sciatic nerve and other gluteal structures of the right side

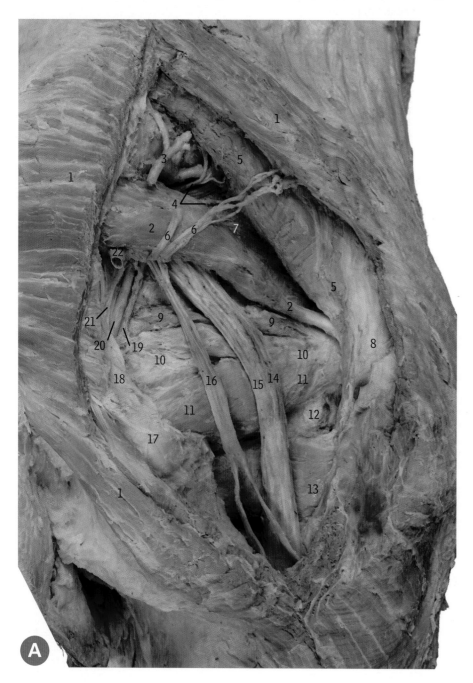

Most of gluteus maximus (1) has been removed (as have the veins that accompany arteries) to show the underlying structures, the most important of which is the sciatic nerve (14 and 15). The key to the region is the piriformis muscle (2): the superior gluteal artery (3) and nerve (4) emerge from the pelvis above piriformis, while all other structures leave the pelvis below piriformis. Apart from the sciatic nerve (14 and 15), these include the inferior gluteal nerve (6) and artery (22) and the posterior femoral cutaneous nerve (16).

 1 Gluteus maximus
 2 Piriformis
 3 Superior gluteal artery
 4 Superior gluteal nerve
 5 Gluteus medius
 6 Inferior gluteal nerve
 7 Gluteus minimus
 8 Greater trochanter of femur
 9 Gemellus superior
10 Obturator internus
11 Gemellus inferior
12 Obturator externus
13 Quadratus femoris
14 Common fibular (*peroneal*) } part of sciatic nerve
15 Tibial
16 Posterior femoral cutaneous nerve
17 Ischial tuberosity
18 Sacrotuberous ligament
19 Nerve to obturator internus
20 Internal pudendal artery
21 Pudendal nerve
22 Inferior gluteal artery

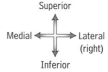

Superior

Medial ⟷ Lateral
(right)

Inferior

Gluteal region
Surface features of the right gluteal region

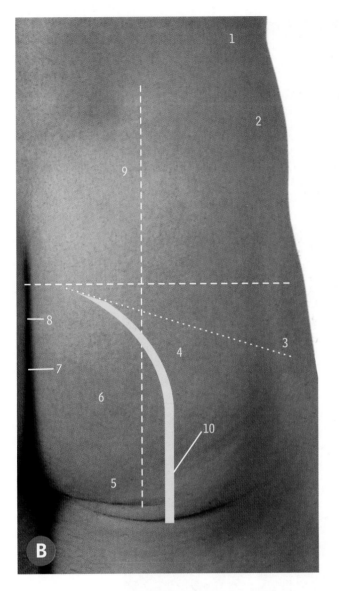

The interrupted lines divide the gluteal region into four quadrants. The surface marking of the lower border of piriformis (the dotted line) is on a line drawn from the midpoint between the posterior superior iliac spine (9) and the coccyx (7) to the top of the greater trochanter of the femur (3). From the midpoint of this line, a curved line (convex laterally) to midway between the ischial tuberosity (6) and the greater trochanter (3) indicates the course of the upper part of the sciatic nerve, indicated here in yellow.

- The superior gluteal nerve runs between gluteus medius and minimus and ends in tensor fasciae latae, supplying all three muscles.

- The inferior gluteal nerve passes straight back into gluteus maximus, supplying that muscle only.

- In the gluteal region the sciatic nerve is a flattened band about 1 cm broad. Its two parts (**A14** and **15**) are usually closely bound together in the gluteal region and the back of the thigh (p. 27, **B10**). In the popliteal fossa at the back of the knee (p. 32, **A**) they separate into the common fibular (*peroneal*) nerve, which supplies the front of the leg and dorsum of the foot, and the tibial nerve, which supplies the back of the leg and sole of the foot.

1 Iliac crest
2 Gluteus medius
3 Greater trochanter of femur
4 Gluteus maximus
5 Fold of buttock
6 Ischial tuberosity
7 Tip of coccyx
8 Natal cleft
9 Posterior superior iliac spine
10 Sciatic nerve

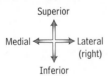

Superior

Medial ⟷ Lateral
(right)

Inferior

Gluteal region *left gluteal region and ischio-anal region, with gluteus maximus and gluteus medius cut through and portions reflected laterally*

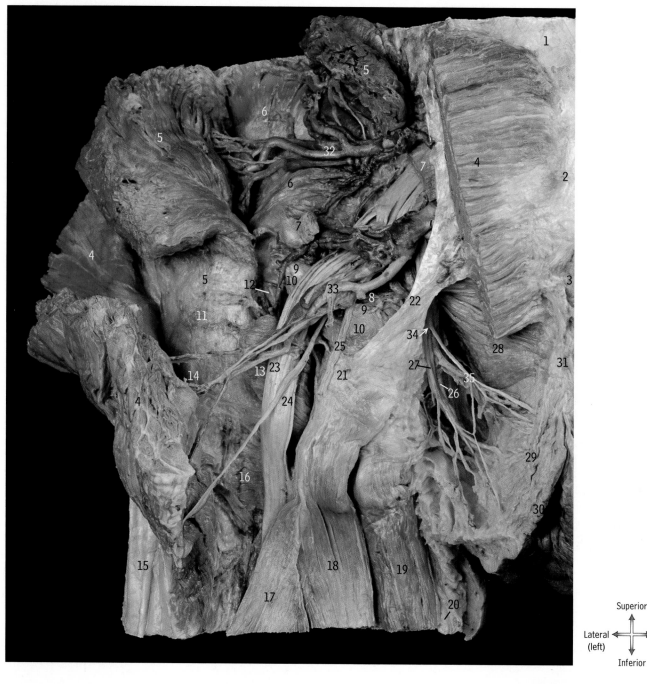

Superior

Lateral ⟷ Medial
(left)

Inferior

1 Posterior layer of lumbar fascia overlying erector spinae	**13** Quadratus femoris	**25** Posterior femoral cutaneous nerve
2 Sacrum	**14** Vastus lateralis	**26** Internal pudendal artery
3 Coccyx	**15** Iliotibial tract	**27** Pudendal nerve
4 Gluteus maximus	**16** Upper part of adductor magnus (adductor minimus)	**28** Levator ani
5 Gluteus medius	**17** Biceps femoris (long head)	**29** External anal sphincter
6 Gluteus minimus	**18** Semitendinosus	**30** Anal margin
7 Piriformis	**19** Adductor magnus	**31** Anococcygeal body
8 Gemellus superior	**20** Gracilis	**32** Superior gluteal artery, vein and nerve
9 Obturator internus	**21** Ischial tuberosity	**33** Inferior gluteal artery, vein and nerve
10 Gemellus inferior	**22** Sacrotuberous ligament	**34** Pudendal canal (arrowed)
11 Greater trochanter of femur	**23** Common fibular (*peroneal*) part of sciatic nerve	**35** Inferior rectal artery, vein and nerve
12 Obturator externus	**24** Tibial part of sciatic nerve	

Gluteal region *right gluteal region and ischio-anal region, with most of gluteus maximus removed*

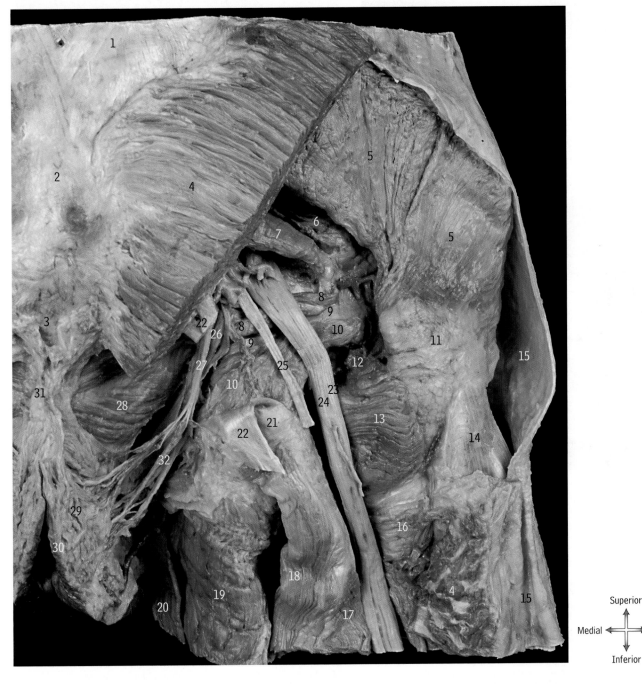

Superior

Medial ←→ Lateral
(right)

Inferior

1   Posterior layer of lumbar fascia overlying erector spinae
2   Sacrum
3   Coccyx
4   Gluteus maximus
5   Gluteus medius
6   Gluteus minimus
7   Piriformis
8   Gemellus superior
9   Obturator internus
10 Gemellus inferior
11 Greater trochanter of femur
12 Obturator externus
13 Quadratus femoris
14 Vastus lateralis
15 Iliotibial tract
16 Upper part of adductor magnus (adductor minimus)
17 Biceps femoris (long head)
18 Semitendinosus
19 Adductor magnus
20 Gracilis
21 Ischial tuberosity
22 Sacrotuberous ligament cut and turned down
23 Common fibular (*peroneal*) part of sciatic nerve
24 Tibial part of sciatic nerve
25 Posterior femoral cutaneous nerve
26 Internal pudendal artery
27 Pudendal nerve
28 Levator ani
29 External anal sphincter
30 Anal margin
31 Anococcygeal body
32 Inferior rectal artery, vein and nerve

Hip joint *left hip bone and femur, with sacrum and coccyx, from the front*

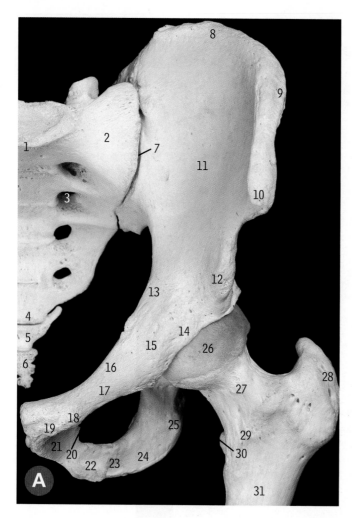

A from the front

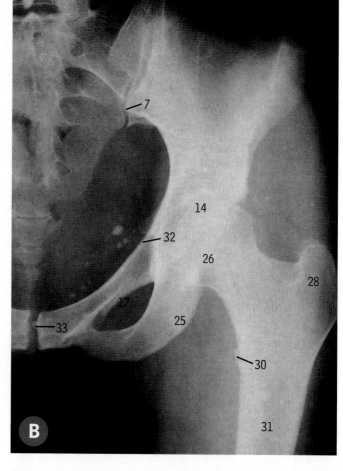

B radiograph. (The translucent areas are gas shadows in the large intestine.)

1 Sacral promontory
2 Ala of sacrum
3 Second anterior sacral foramen, for anterior ramus of S2 nerve
4 Apex of sacrum
5 First coccygeal vertebra, with transverse process
6 Fused coccygeal vertebrae
7 Sacroiliac joint
8 Iliac crest, palpable throughout its whole length, and a possible site (like the sternum) for bone marrow biopsy
9 Tubercle of iliac crest
10 Anterior superior iliac spine, for inguinal ligament and sartorius
11 Iliac fossa, a term also applied to the lower lateral region of the anterior abdominal wall
12 Anterior inferior iliac spine, for part of rectus femoris
13 Arcuate line of ilium, forming part of the pelvic brim
14 Rim of acetabulum, the socket for the head of the femur (**26**)
15 Iliopubic eminence, site of union between ilium and superior ramus of the pubis (**17**)
16 Pectineal line (pecten) of pubis
17 Superior ramus of pubis

18 Pubic tubercle, a palpable landmark
19 Pubic crest, for rectus abdominis
20 Obturator foramen
21 Body of pubis
22 Inferior ramus of pubis
23 Site of union of pubic and ischial rami (**22** and **24**)
24 Ramus of ischium
25 Ischial tuberosity, best seen from behind (C, **16**)
26 Head of femur
27 Neck, the part of the femur most commonly fractured
28 Greater trochanter. Gluteus medius and minimus are attached to its front and lateral side
29 Intertrochanteric line, for the capsule of the hip joint and not to be confused with the intertrochanteric crest on the back of the bone (C, **23**)
30 Tip of lesser trochanter, best seen from behind (C, **25**)
31 Shaft of femur
32 Ischial spine
33 Pubic symphysis

C *Left bone and femur, with sacrum and coccyx, from behind*

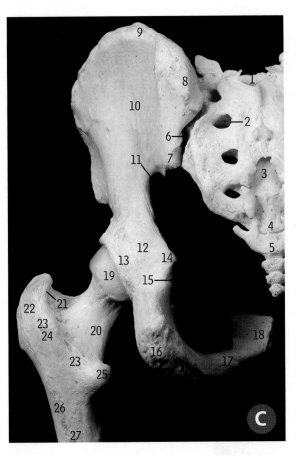

1 Sacral canal
2 Second posterior sacral foramen, for posterior ramus of S2 nerve
3 Sacral hiatus, the lower opening of the sacral canal and here unusually high
4 Apex of sacrum
5 First coccygeal vertebra, with below it the fused second to fourth coccygeal vertebrae
6 Sacroiliac joint
7 Posterior inferior iliac spine
8 Posterior superior iliac spine
9 Iliac crest
10 Ilium, outer surface
11 Greater sciatic notch
12 Site of fusion of ilium and ischium
13 Rim of acetabulum, the socket which receives the head of the femur (**19**)
14 Ischial spine, separating the greater and lesser sciatic notches (**11** and **15**)
15 Lesser sciatic notch
16 Ischial tuberosity, which bears the weight when sitting
17 Ramus of ischium joining inferior ramus of pubis
18 Body of pubis
19 Head of femur, making the hip joint with the acetabulum of the hip bone (**13**)
20 Neck, labeled along the site of attachment of the capsule of the hip joint, which does not extend as far as the intertrochanteric crest (**23**)
21 Trochanteric fossa for obturator externus
22 Greater tuberosity whose curved upper margin receives piriformis and obturator internus
23 Intertrochanteric crest
24 Quadrate tubercle, for quadratus femoris
25 Lesser trochanter, for psoas major with fibers from iliacus just below it
26 Gluteal tuberosity, receiving part of the attachment of gluteus maximus (the rest is attached to the fascia lata, the deep fascia of the thigh)
27 Shaft of femur

C
Superior
Lateral ⟷ Medial
(left)
Inferior

D *Left hip joint capsule (male), from the front, with all surrounding muscles removed except for obturator externus*

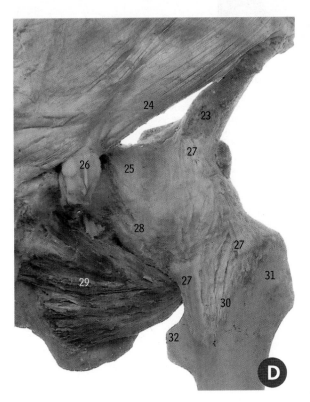
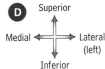

23 Anterior inferior iliac spine
24 Inguinal ligament
25 Iliopubic eminence
26 Spermatic cord
27 Iliofemoral ligament, like an inverted V, reinforcing and blending with the front of the capsule
28 Pubofemoral ligament, reinforcing and blending with the more medial part of the capsule
29 Obturator externus
30 Intertrochanteric line
31 Greater trochanter
32 Lesser trochanter

D
Superior
Medial ⟷ Lateral
(left)
Inferior

Hip joint *axial section through the left hip joint at the level of the last, fifth segment of the sacrum, from below*

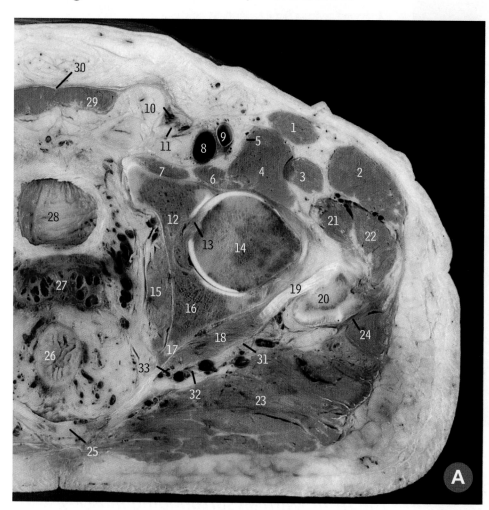

1 Sartorius
2 Tensor fasciae latae
3 Rectus femoris
4 Iliacus
5 Femoral nerve
6 Psoas major
7 Pectineus
8 Femoral vein
9 Femoral artery
10 Spermatic cord
11 Vas deferens
12 Acetabulum (pubic portion)
13 Ligamentum teres
14 Femoral head
15 Obturator internus
16 Ischium
17 Ischial spine
18 Gemellus superior
19 Obturator internus tendon
20 Greater trochanter
21 Gluteus minimus
22 Gluteus medius
23 Gluteus maximus
24 Trochanteric bursa
25 Sacrum fifth segment
26 Rectum
27 Seminal vesicle
28 Bladder
29 Rectus abdominis
30 Linea alba
31 Sciatic nerve
32 Inferior gluteal artery and vein
33 Pudendal nerve and internal pudendal artery and vein

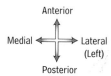

Anterior
Medial — Lateral (Left)
Posterior

A

Muscles producing movements at the hip joint consist of the following:

- **Flexion** (moving the thigh forward and upward toward the abdomen): psoas and iliacus, with rectus femoris, sartorius, tensor fasciae latae, pectineus, adductor longus and adductor brevis.

- **Extension** (moving the thigh backward): gluteus maximus, semimembranosus, semitendinosus, long head of biceps and ischial part of adductor magnus.

- **Abduction** (moving the thigh laterally away from the midline): gluteus medius, gluteus minimus, with tensor fasciae latae and piriformis.

- **Adduction** (moving the thigh medially toward the midline): adductor longus, adductor brevis, adductor magnus, pectineus, gracilis and quadratus femoris.

- **Medial rotation** (rotating the thigh inward in the long axis of the limb): anterior fibres of gluteus medius and gluteus minimus, with tensor fasciae latae. (Electromyography does not support the long-held view that psoas major is a medial rotator.)

- **Lateral rotation** (rotating the thigh outward in the long axis of the limb): obturator externus, obturator internus and gemelli, piriformis, quadratus femoris, gluteus maximus and sartorius.

- The coronal section of the joint in **C** demonstrates the thickness of the capsule (**15**) but does not of course show the ligaments that reinforce the outside of the capsule (iliofemoral at the front, and pubofemoral and ischiofemoral below and behind).

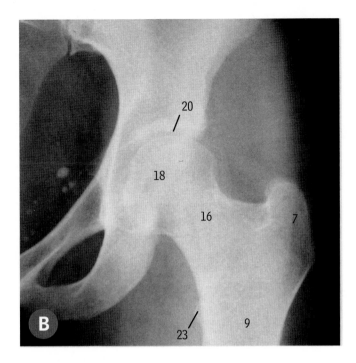

B radiograph

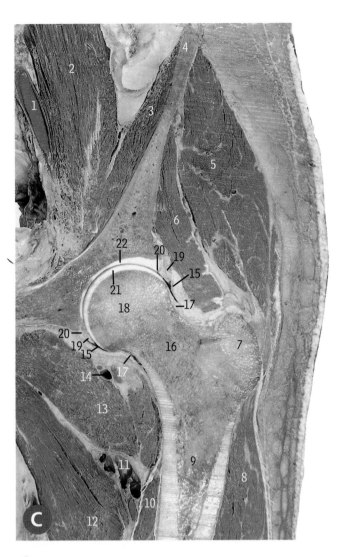

C coronal section of the left hip joint, from the front

1   External iliac artery
2   Psoas major
3   Iliacus
4   Iliac crest
5   Gluteus medius
6   Gluteus minimus
7   Greater trochanter of femur
8   Vastus lateralis
9   Shaft of femur
10 Vastus medialis
11 Profunda femoris vessels
12 Adductor longus
13 Pectineus
14 Medial circumflex femoral
    vessels
15 Capsule of hip joint
16 Neck of femur
17 Zona orbicularis of capsule
18 Head of femur
19 Acetabular labrum
20 Rim of acetabulum
21 Hyaline cartilage of head
    of femur
22 Hyaline cartilage of
    acetabulum
23 Lesser trochanter of femur

B **C**   Superior
Medial ⟷ Lateral
(Left)
Inferior

The head of the femur (18) sits in the hip bone's acetabulum (20), which is deepened at the periphery by the fibrous acetabular labrum (19). Note the hyaline cartilage on the joint surfaces (21 and 22), and the capsule (15) whose circular fibers (zona orbicularis, 17) keep it close to the neck of the femur (16). Gluteus medius (5) and gluteus minimus (6) converge on to the greater trochanter (7), and below the head and neck of the femur (18 and 16), the tendon of psoas major (2) and some muscle fibres of iliacus (3) are passing backward to reach the lesser trochanter on the back of the bone. Compare major features in the section with the radiograph.

Thigh, Knee and Leg

2

Thigh *front of the right upper thigh*

Part of the fascia lata (deep fascia of the thigh, 14) has been removed to display the femoral vessels and nerve and the adjacent muscles. The femoral nerve (21), artery (20), vein (18) and canal (17) lie in that order from lateral to medial beneath the inguinal ligament (19). The great saphenous vein (12) passes through the saphenous opening (16) in the fascia lata to enter the femoral vein (18); a number of smaller veins enter the great saphenous just before it joins the femoral.

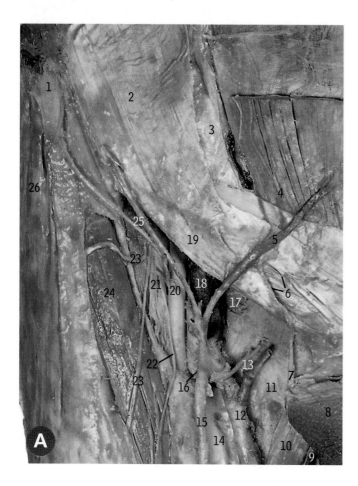

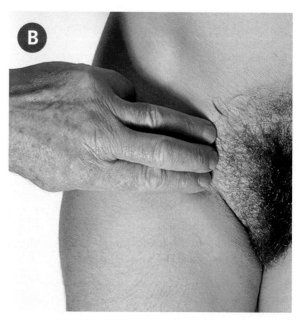

Ⓐ **inguinal and femoral regions, in the female**

Ⓑ **palpation of femoral pulse**

- The femoral pulse can be felt midway between the anterior superior iliac spine and the midline pubic symphysis (the midinguinal point or femoral point).

Ⓐ Ⓑ Superior
Lateral ⟷ Medial
(right)
Inferior

- Various superficial veins (**5, 13, 15, 25**) run into the great saphenous vein (**12**); this helps to distinguish the great saphenous from the femoral vein (**18**), which superficially at this level receives only the great saphenous itself. See p. 70 for further details of the great saphenous vein.

- Although arising at the *front* of the thigh, the profunda femoris artery is the main supply to muscles on the *back* of the thigh as well as those on the front.

- The adductor canal, which is triangular in cross section, is bounded in front by sartorius, laterally by vastus medialis, and behind by adductor longus (above) and adductor magnus (below). The contents of the adductor canal are the femoral artery and vein, the saphenous nerve and the nerve to vastus medialis.

1   Anterior superior iliac spine
2   External oblique aponeurosis
3   Cut edge of rectus sheath
4   Rectus abdominis
5   Superficial epigastric vein
6   Superficial inguinal ring
7   Round ligament of uterus
8   Mons pubis
9   Gracilis
10 Adductor longus
11 Pectineus
12 Great saphenous vein
13 Superficial external pudendal vessels
14 Fascia lata
15 Accessory saphenous vein
16 Lower edge of saphenous opening
17 Position of femoral canal
18 Femoral vein
19 Inguinal ligament
20 Femoral artery
21 Femoral nerve
22 Medial   ⎫
23 Intermediate ⎬ femoral cutaneous nerve
             ⎭
24 Sartorius
25 Superficial circumflex iliac vessels
26 Fascia lata overlying tensor fasciae latae

Thigh *front of the right upper thigh (male)*

In this deeper dissection the removal of part of sartorius (3) displays the profunda femoris artery (24). The femoral artery (9) passes in front of adductor longus (18); the profunda (24) passes behind it. Separation of the adjacent borders of pectineus (13) and adductor longus (18) allows the anterior division of the obturator nerve (15) to be seen in front of adductor brevis (17). The medial circumflex femoral artery (12) disappears backward between pectineus (13) and the tendon of psoas (hidden behind the uppermost part of the femoral artery (upper 9). The lateral circumflex femoral artery (11, which often arises directly from the femoral artery, as here, and not from the profunda) courses laterally and supplies adjacent muscles. Branches of the femoral nerve (8) include the saphenous nerve (25), which will run as far as the medial side of the foot.

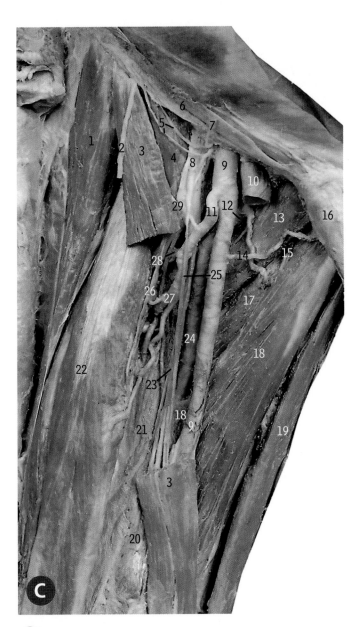

1	Tensor fasciae latae
2	Lateral femoral cutaneous nerve
3	Sartorius
4	Iliacus
5	Superficial circumflex iliac artery (double)
6	Inguinal ligament
7	Superficial epigastric artery
8	Femoral nerve
9	Femoral artery
10	Femoral vein
11	Lateral circumflex femoral artery
12	Medial circumflex femoral artery
13	Pectineus
14	Superficial external pudendal artery
15	Anterior branch of obturator nerve
16	Spermatic cord
17	Adductor brevis
18	Adductor longus
19	Gracilis
20	Vastus medialis
21	Vastus intermedius
22	Rectus femoris
23	Nerve to vastus medialis
24	Profunda femoris artery
25	Saphenous nerve
26	Nerve to rectus femoris
27	Descending ⎫ branch of lateral circumflex
28	Transverse ⎬ femoral artery
29	Ascending ⎭

Superior

Lateral (right) ←→ Medial

Inferior

C femoral vessels and nerve, in the male

Thigh *lower right thigh, medial side*

The lower part of sartorius (3) has been displaced medially to open up the lower part of the adductor canal and expose the femoral artery (4) passing through the opening in adductor magnus (6) to enter the popliteal fossa behind the knee and become the popliteal artery.

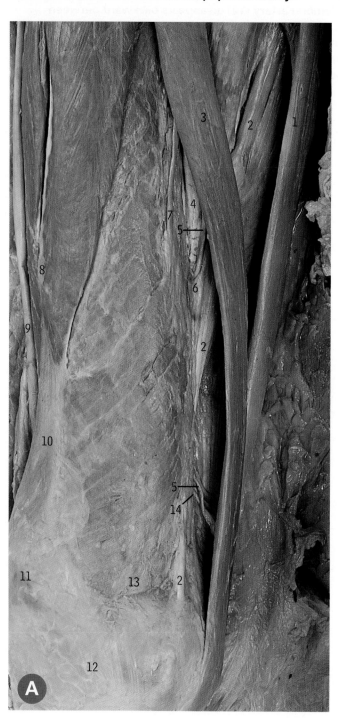

1   Gracilis
2   Adductor magnus
3   Sartorius
4   Femoral artery
5   Saphenous nerve
6   Opening in adductor magnus
7   Vastus medialis and nerve
8   Rectus femoris
9   Iliotibial tract
10 Quadriceps tendon
11 Patella
12 Medial patellar retinaculum
13 Lowest (horizontal) fibres of vastus medialis
14 Saphenous branch of descending genicular artery

Superior
(proximal)

Lateral ←——→ Medial
(left)

Inferior
(distal)

Ⓐ   from the front and medial side

Thigh *axial section through lower right thigh*

The section is viewed as when looking upward from knee to hip. The three vastus muscles **(1, 3, 5)** envelop the femur **(2)** at the front and sides, and rectus femoris **(4)** at this level is narrow and is becoming tendinous. The femoral vessels **(20)** are between vastus medialis **(1)** and adductor magnus **(12)**, approaching the adductor magnus opening **(13)**, and the profunda femoris vessels **(11)** lie close to the back of the femur **(2)**. The sciatic nerve **(10)** is deeply placed between biceps **(8, 9)** laterally and semimembranosus **(14)** and semitendinosus **(15)** medially.

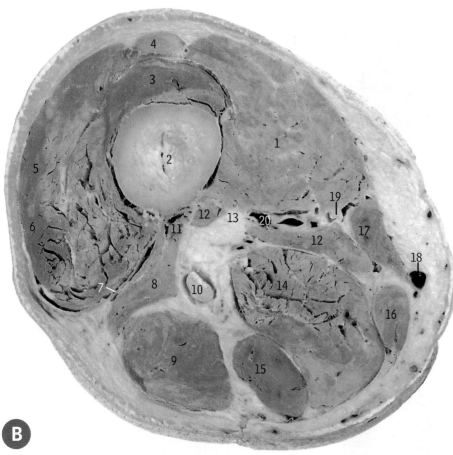

1	Vastus medialis
2	Femur
3	Vastus intermedius
4	Rectus femoris
5	Vastus lateralis
6	Iliotibial tract
7	Lateral intermuscular septum
8	Short head of biceps
9	Long head of biceps
10	Sciatic nerve
11	Profunda femoris vessels
12	Adductor magnus
13	Opening in adductor magnus
14	Semimembranosus
15	Semitendinosus
16	Gracilis
17	Sartorius
18	Great saphenous vein
19	Saphenous nerve
20	Femoral vessels

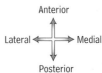

Anterior

Lateral ←——→ Medial

Posterior

B

B axial section at the level of the opening in adductor magnus

- The muscles commonly called the hamstrings span both the hip and knee joints: they arise from the ischial tuberosity and run to the upper end of the tibia and fibula, and consist of semitendinosus, semimembranosus, and the long head of biceps. The short head of biceps is not a hamstring, since although it joins the long head it arises from the back of the femur and hence does not span the hip joint. Semitendinosus is named from the long tendon at its lower end. Semimembranosus is named from the broad tendinous origin at its upper end.

Knee joint *left knee joint*

Flexion of the knee, as in **B**, exposes a much larger area of the femoral condyles (**4, 7**) than is seen in extension (as in **A** and **C**). In **B** the medial and lateral menisci (**18, 22**) lie between the condyles of the femur and tibia (**4, 9; 7, 12**), with the anterior cruciate ligament (**19**) passing backward and laterally from the upper surface of the tibia to the medial surface of the lateral condyle of the femur. Compare the MR image in **C** with the dissection in **B**.

In **D** the joint has been opened up by cutting through the quadriceps muscle (**26**) and the patellar ligament (**30**), and turning laterally the large flap which includes the patella (**28**), in order to show the joint cavity from the front and the margins of the suprapatellar bursa (**27**) which is in direct continuity with the cavity of the knee joint.

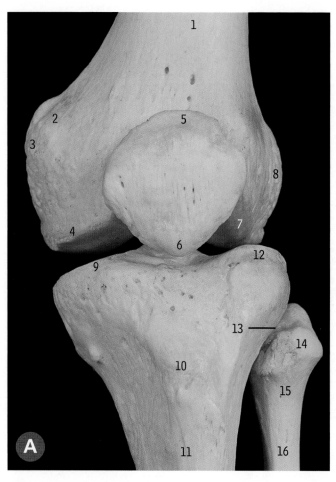

A bones, with the knee joint in extension, from the front

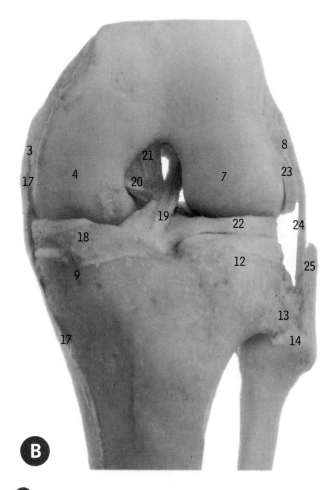

B bones and ligaments, with the knee joint in flexion and the patella removed, from the front

- The **lateral ligament** (**B24**, properly called the fibular collateral ligament) is a rounded cord about 5 cm long, passing from the lateral epicondyle of the femur (**B8**) to the head of the fibula (**B14**).

- The **medial ligament** (**B17**, properly called the tibial collateral ligament) is a broad flat band about 12 cm long passing from the medial epicondyle of the femur (**B3**) to the medial side of the medial condyle of the tibia (**B9**) and to an extensive area of the medial surface below the condyle. At the side it fuses with the medial meniscus (**B18**; see also p. 30, **B18** and **19**); the lateral ligament (**B24**) does not fuse with the lateral meniscus (**B22**), to which the tendon of popliteus has an attachment (p. 30, **C28**).

- For notes on the cruciate ligaments and menisci see p. 30.

1 Shaft of femur
2 Adductor tubercle
3 Medial epicondyle
4 Medial condyle
5 Base of patella
6 Apex of patella
7 Lateral condyle
8 Lateral epicondyle
9 Medial condyle of tibia
10 Tibial tuberosity
11 Shaft
12 Lateral condyle
13 Superior tibiofibular joint (with capsule in **B**)
14 Head ⎫
15 Neck ⎬ of fibula
16 Shaft ⎭

17 Medial ligament
18 Medial meniscus
19 Anterior cruciate ligament
20 Anterior meniscofemoral ligament
21 Posterior cruciate ligament
22 Lateral meniscus
23 Popliteus tendon
24 Lateral ligament
25 Biceps tendon
26 Quadriceps femoris
27 Margins of suprapatellar bursa
28 Posterior surface of patella
29 Infrapatellar fat pad
30 Patellar ligament
31 Deep infrapatellar bursa

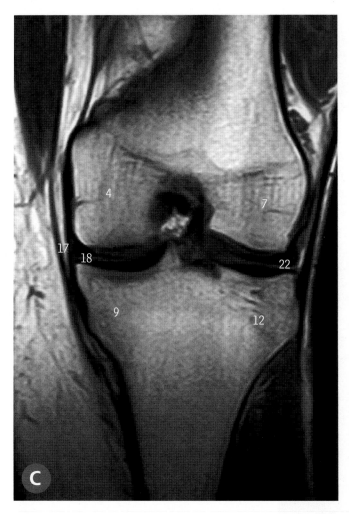

C coronal magnetic resonance image (MRI)

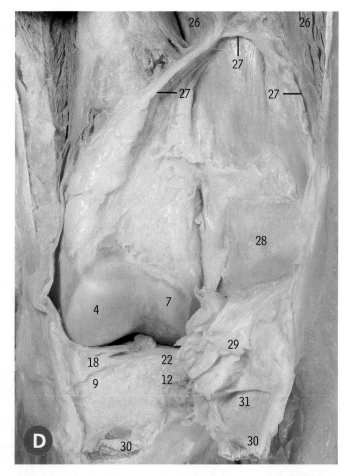

D opened up from the front, with the knee joint in extension and the patella turned laterally

Superior
(proximal)

Medial ⟷ Lateral
(left)

Inferior
(distal)

A **B** **C** and **D**

Knee joint *left knee joint*

The joint in **B** is partly flexed, showing less of the articular surfaces of the femoral condyles (**4, 6**) than in **A**. In **B** the posterior cruciate ligament (**20**) spills over onto the uppermost part of the posterior surface of the tibia. The attachment of the medial meniscus (**19**) to the medial ligament (**18**) is clearly seen; the lateral meniscus (**23**) has no attachment to the lateral ligament (**24**) but gives rise to the posterior meniscofemoral ligament (**22**) which lies on the surface of the posterior cruciate ligament (**20**), here obscuring the anterior meniscofemoral ligament (**27**).

The view in C demonstrates the shapes of the medial and lateral menisci (**19, 23**), the tibial attachments of the anterior and posterior cruciate ligaments (**21, 20**) and the anterior and posterior meniscofemoral ligaments (**27, 22**) which pass respectively in front of and behind the posterior cruciate ligament (**20**).

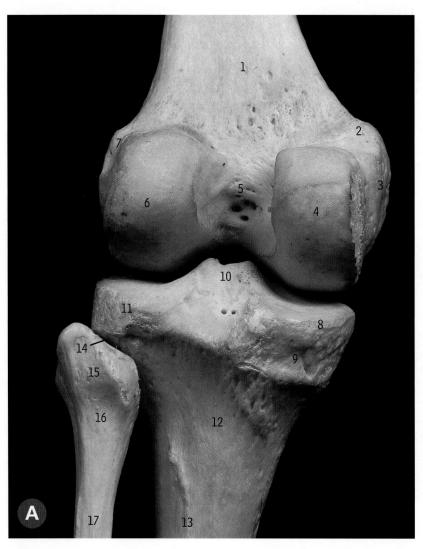

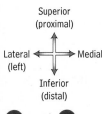

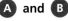

1 Popliteal surface of femur
2 Adductor tubercle
3 Medial epicondyle
4 Medial condyle
5 Intercondylar fossa
6 Lateral condyle
7 Lateral epicondyle
8 Medial condyle of tibia
9 Groove for semimembranosus insertion
10 Intercondylar eminence
11 Lateral condyle
12 Popliteal surface of tibia
13 Soleal line
14 Superior tibiofibular joint (with capsule in **B**)
15 Head of fibula ⎫
16 Neck   ⎬ of fibula
17 Shaft   ⎭
18 Medial ligament
19 Medial meniscus
20 Posterior cruciate ligament
21 Anterior cruciate ligament
22 Posterior meniscofemoral ligament
23 Lateral meniscus (with marker under medial margin in **C**)
24 Lateral ligament
25 Popliteus tendon
26 Biceps tendon
27 Anterior meniscofemoral ligament
28 Attachment of popliteus to lateral meniscus

Superior
(proximal)

Lateral ←——→ Medial
(left)

Inferior
(distal)

A and **B**

A bones, from behind

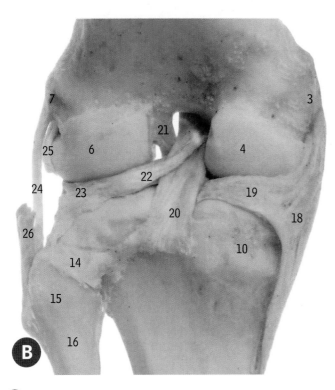

B ligaments, from behind

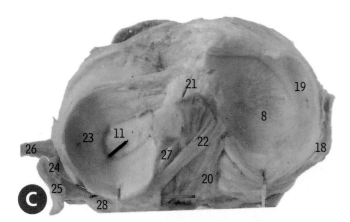

C upper surface of tibia with ligaments, from above

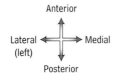

Anterior

Lateral ⟷ Medial
(left)

Posterior

- The cruciate ligaments are named from their attachments to the tibia.

- The anterior cruciate ligament (**C21**), from the front of the upper surface of the tibia, passes upward, backward and laterally to become attached to the medial side of the lateral condyle of the femur (p. 28, **B19**).

- The posterior cruciate ligament (**C20**), from the back of the upper surface and the very top of the posterior surface of the tibia, passes upward, forward and medially to become attached to lateral side of the medial condyle of the femur (p. 28, **B21**).

- The anterior and posterior meniscofemoral ligaments (**C27**, **C22**) arise from the back of the lateral meniscus and run upward and forward like a two-pronged fork embracing the posterior cruciate ligament (**C20**) at its front and back and fusing with it.

- The C-shaped fibrocartilaginous menisci (**C19** and **C23**) are attached by their ends (the horns of the menisci) to the intercondylar area of the upper surface of the tibia.

- Muscles producing movements at the knee joint include the following:

  Flexion (bending the leg backwards): semimembranosus, semitendinosus, biceps, gracilis, sartorius, gastrocnemius and popliteus.

  Extension (straightening the flexed knee): vastus medialis, vastus intermedius, vastus lateralis, rectus femoris, and tensor fasciae latae and gluteus maximus acting via the iliotibial tract.

  Medial rotation *of the flexed leg* (rotating the leg medially in the long axis of the leg): semimembranosus, semitendinosus, gracilis, sartorius and popliteus.

  Lateral rotation *of the flexed leg* (rotating the leg laterally in the long axis of the leg): biceps.

- Because of the shape of the articulating surfaces and the tension in the ligaments, there is some medial rotation of the femur on the tibia towards the end of extension (assuming the tibia to be fixed); this is the so-called 'locking of the knee joint'. To begin flexion, popliteus 'unlocks' the joint by causing some lateral rotation of the femur on the tibia (assuming the tibia to be fixed); the other flexors can then carry on the movement.

Knee joint *popliteal fossa and back of the knee*

In A the fascia that forms the roof of the fossa and the fat within it have been removed. At the upper part of the fossa, biceps (10) is on the lateral side with the common fibular (*peroneal*) nerve (9) at its posterior border, and semimembranosus (3) with semitendinosus (4) overlying it are on the medial side. At the lower part of the fossa, the medial head of gastrocnemius (15) is on the medial side, while on the lateral side plantaris (11) lies just above the lateral head of gastrocnemius (12). Of the principal structures within the fossa, the tibial nerve (7) is the most superficial, with the popliteal vein (6) behind it and the popliteal artery (5) deep to the vein.

In the lateral view in B, the ridge formed by the iliotibial tract (18) lies above (anterior to) the tendon of biceps (10), at the lateral boundary of the popliteal fossa (25). Below the head of the fibula (24) the common fibular (*peroneal*) nerve (9) is palpable and can be rolled against the neck of the bone.

1 Sartorius
2 Gracilis
3 Semimembranosus
4 Semitendinosus
5 Popliteal artery
6 Popliteal vein
7 Tibial nerve
8 Lateral cutaneous nerve of calf
9 Common fibular (*peroneal*) nerve
10 Biceps
11 Plantaris
12 Lateral head of gastrocnemius
13 Small saphenous vein (double)
14 Sural nerve
15 Medial head of gastrocnemius
16 Nerve to medial head ⎫
17 Nerve to lateral head ⎬ of gastrocnemius
18 Iliotibial tract
19 Patella
20 Margin of lateral condyle of femur
21 Patellar ligament
22 Tuberosity of tibia
23 Margin of lateral condyle of tibia
24 Head of fibula
25 Popliteal fossa

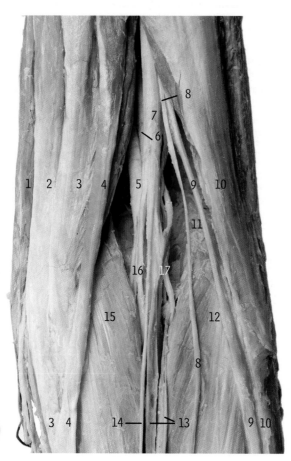
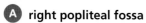

A right popliteal fossa

Superior
(proximal)

Medial ⬌ Lateral
(right)

Inferior
(distal)

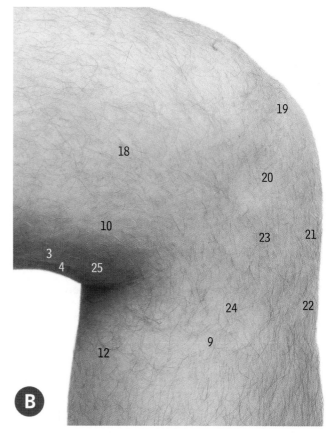

B surface landmarks of the flexed right knee, from the lateral side

Superior
(proximal)

Posterior ⬌ Anterior

Inferior
(distal)

Knee joint *popliteal fossa and back of the knee*

Most of gastrocnemius, soleus and other muscles have been removed to display popliteus (**6**) and the posterior surface of the knee joint capsule (**13**), which is reinforced by the tendinous fibers of semimembranosus (**11**) that form the oblique popliteal ligament (**12**).

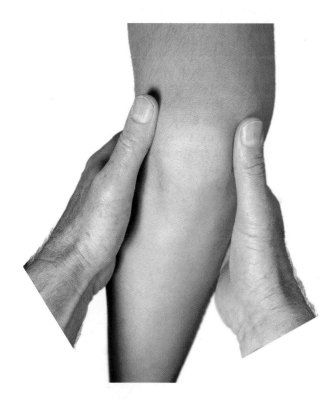

C palpation of the right popliteal pulse

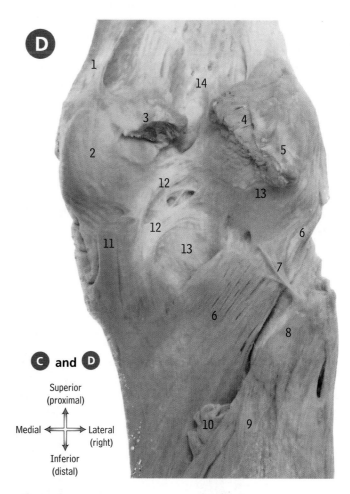

C and **D**

Superior
(proximal)

Medial ← → Lateral
(right)

Inferior
(distal)

D right popliteus muscle and knee joint capsule, from behind

- The deep position of the popliteal artery (**A5**)—deep to the popliteal vein (**A6**), which in turn is deep to the tibial nerve (**A7**)—makes feeling the popliteal pulse difficult. It is best felt from the front, grasping the sides of the knee with both hands, placing the thumbs beside the patella and pressing the tips of the fingers deeply into the midline of the fossa.

- The slender arcuate popliteal ligament (**D7**) arches over popliteus (**D6**) as it enters the joint capsule to reach the lateral side of the lateral condyle of the femur.

---

1 Adductor magnus
2 Capsule overlying medial condyle of femur
3 Medial head of gastrocnemius
4 Plantaris
5 Lateral head of gastrocnemius
6 Popliteus
7 Arcuate popliteal ligament
8 Head of fibula
9 Soleus
10 Popliteal vessels and tibial nerve
11 Semimembranosus
12 Oblique popliteal ligament
13 Capsule of knee joint
14 Popliteal surface of femur

Leg and foot survey
Muscles and superficial vessels and nerves of the left leg and foot

Skin, subcutaneous tissue and most of the deep fascia have been removed, and different aspects of the same specimen are shown. Lateral to the medial (subcutaneous) surface (**A2**) and anterior border of the tibia is the largest muscle of the front of the leg, tibialis anterior (**A6, C6**), which becomes tendinous in the lower part of the leg and has the tendons of extensor hallucis longus (**A7**) and extensor digitorum longus (**A8**) lateral to it. On the medial side the bulk of gastrocnemius (**A3, B3**) and the underlying soleus (**A4**) overlie the flexor muscles whose tendons pass behind the medial malleolus (**B9**) — tibialis posterior (**B19**), flexor digitorum longus (**B18**) and flexor hallucis longus (**B16**), in that order from front to back. On the lateral side, fibularis (*peroneus*) longus (**C23**) largely overlies fibularis (*peroneus*) brevis (**C25**); their tendons pass behind the lateral malleolus (**C10**). At the back gastrocnemius (**D3**) has been detached at its upper end to show the underlying soleus (**E4**), which in turn has been detached with plantaris (**E31**) in **F** to display the underlying flexor muscle — tibialis posterior (**F19**), the deepest muscle, which is overlapped by flexor hallucis longus (**F16**) on the lateral side and flexor digitorum longus (**F18**) on the medial side.

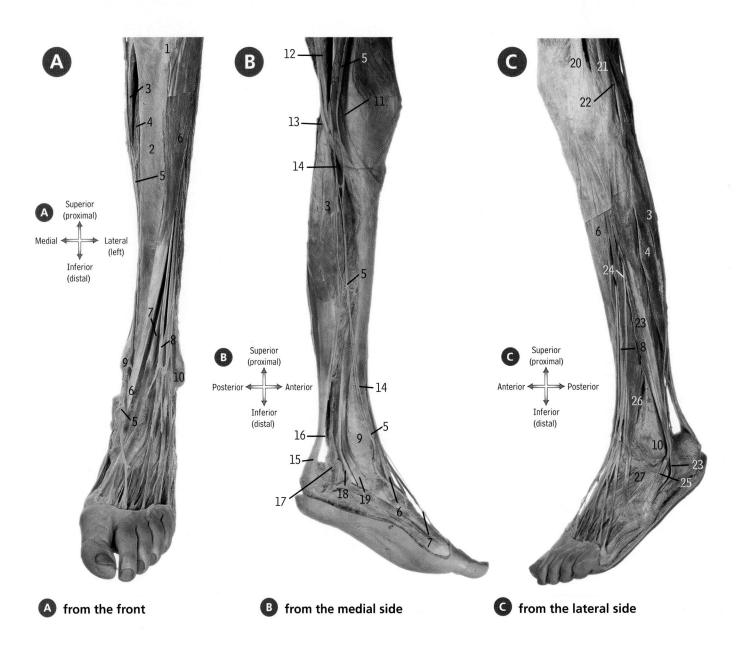

A from the front   **B** from the medial side   **C** from the lateral side

1 Patellar ligament (lower edge)
2 Medial surface of tibia
3 Gastrocnemius
4 Soleus
5 Great saphenous vein
6 Tibialis anterior
7 Extensor hallucis longus
8 Extensor digitorum longus
9 Medial malleolus
10 Lateral malleolus
11 Sartorius
12 Gracilis
13 Semitendinosus
14 Saphenous nerve
15 Tendo calcaneus
16 Flexor hallucis longus
17 Tibial nerve and posterior tibial vessels

18 Flexor digitorum longus
19 Tibialis posterior
20 Iliotibial tract
21 Biceps femoris
22 Common fibular (*peroneal*) nerve
23 Fibularis (*peroneus*) longus
24 Superficial fibular (*peroneal*) nerve
25 Fibularis (*peroneus*) brevis
26 Fibularis (*peroneus*) tertius
27 Extensor digitorum brevis
28 Semimembranosus
29 Small saphenous vein
30 Sural nerve
31 Plantaris
32 Tibial nerve
33 Popliteal vein overlying artery
34 Fascia over popliteus

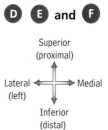

Superior
(proximal)

Lateral ←→ Medial
(left)

Inferior
(distal)

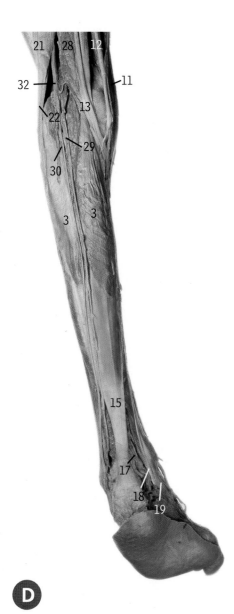

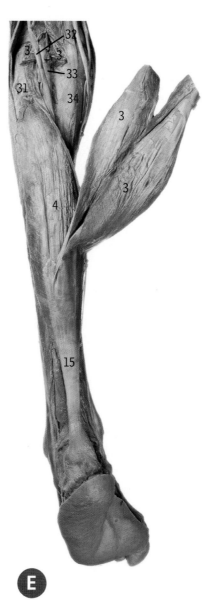

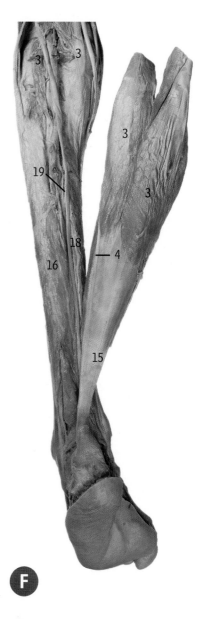

D from behind

E from behind, with
gastrocnemius detached

F from behind, with
gastrocnemius, plantaris
and soleus detached

Foot

3

Surface landmarks of the foot *surface landmarks of the left foot*

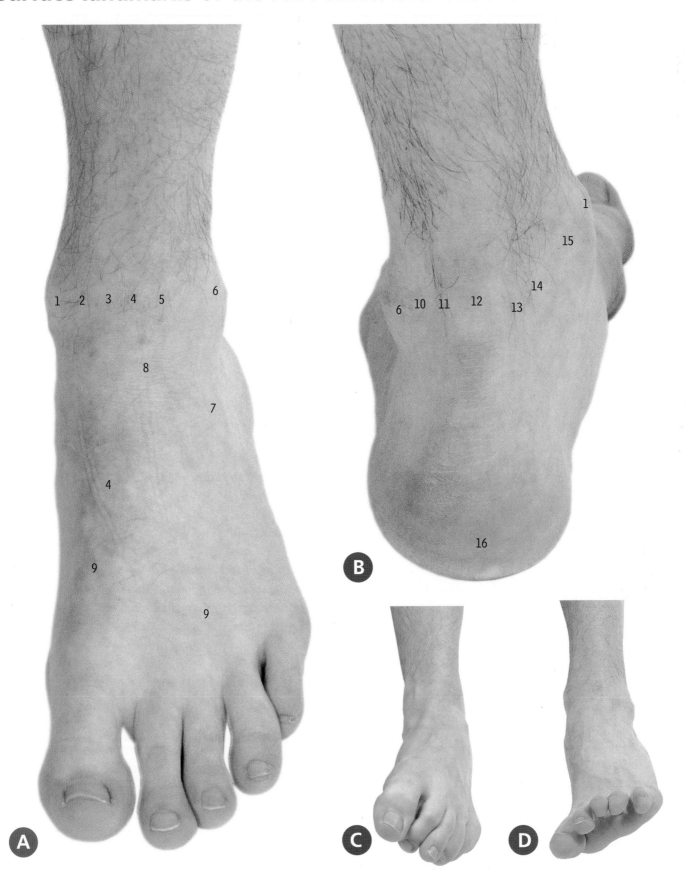

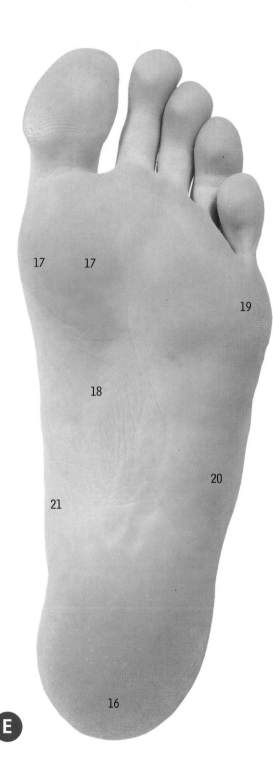

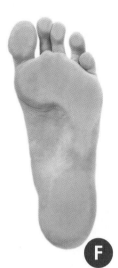

1 Medial malleolus
2 Great saphenous vein and saphenous nerve
3 Tibialis anterior
4 Extensor hallucis longus
5 Extensor digitorum longus
6 Lateral malleolus
7 Extensor digitorum brevis
8 Dorsalis pedis artery
9 Dorsal venous arch
10 Fibularis (*peroneus*) longus and brevis
11 Small saphenous vein and sural nerve
12 Tendo calcaneus
13 Flexor hallucis longus
14 Posterior tibial artery and tibial nerve
15 Flexor digitorum longus and tibialis posterior
16 Tuberosity of calcaneus
17 Sesamoid bones under head of first metatarsal
18 Base of first metatarsal
19 Head of fifth metatarsal
20 Tuberosity of base of fifth metatarsal
21 Tuberosity of navicular

Definitions of movements are as follows:

- **Extension:** from the Latin for straightening out, but as far as the ankle and foot are concerned it means bending the foot and/or toes upwards, and is also known as dorsiflexion.

- **Flexion:** from the Latin for bending. In the ankle and foot it means bending the foot and/or toes downwards, which is also known as plantarflexion.

- **Abduction:** from the Latin for moving away. In the foot it means spreading the toes apart (the corresponding movement of the fingers is much more extensive).

- **Adduction:** from the Latin for moving towards. In the foot it means drawing the toes together.

- **Inversion:** from the Latin for turning in — turning the foot so that the sole faces more inwards (medially).

- **Eversion:** from the Latin for turning out — moving the foot so that the sole faces more outwards (laterally) (a more limited movement than inversion).

For further details see pp. 87 and 99.

A from the front and above (dorsal surface, dorsum)

B from behind

C from the front, in inversion

D from the front, in eversion with abduction of toes

E from below (plantar surface, sole)

F imprint of sole when weight-bearing (viewed through a glass plate)

Surface landmarks of the left foot

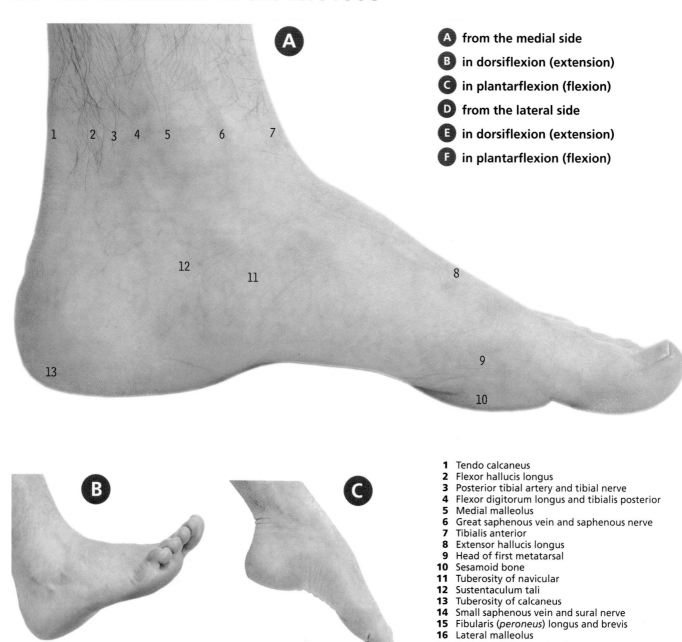

Ⓐ from the medial side

Ⓑ in dorsiflexion (extension)

Ⓒ in plantarflexion (flexion)

Ⓓ from the lateral side

Ⓔ in dorsiflexion (extension)

Ⓕ in plantarflexion (flexion)

1 Tendo calcaneus
2 Flexor hallucis longus
3 Posterior tibial artery and tibial nerve
4 Flexor digitorum longus and tibialis posterior
5 Medial malleolus
6 Great saphenous vein and saphenous nerve
7 Tibialis anterior
8 Extensor hallucis longus
9 Head of first metatarsal
10 Sesamoid bone
11 Tuberosity of navicular
12 Sustentaculum tali
13 Tuberosity of calcaneus
14 Small saphenous vein and sural nerve
15 Fibularis (*peroneus*) longus and brevis
16 Lateral malleolus
17 Extensor digitorum brevis
18 Extensor digitorum longus
19 Tuberosity of base of fifth metatarsal
20 Head of fifth metatarsal

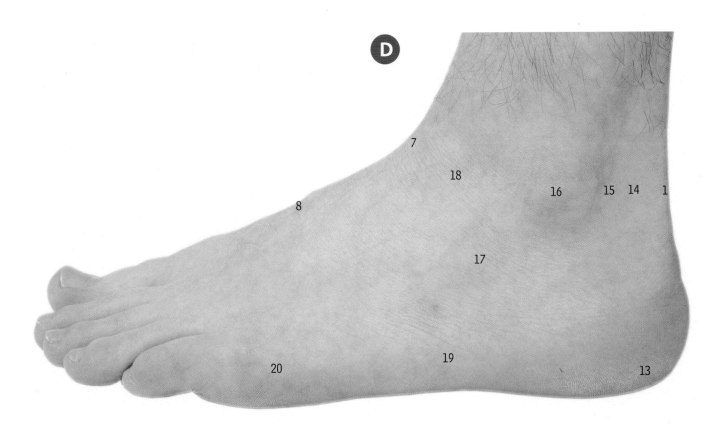

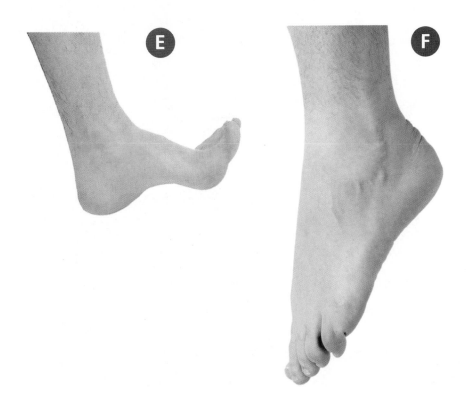

- Pulsation in the dorsalis pedis artery (p. 78, 14) is normally palpable between the tendons of extensor hallucis longus (8) and extensor digitorum longus (18), on a line from the midpoint between the medial and lateral malleoli to the proximal end of the first intermetatarsal space. However, the artery is absent in about 12% of feet (see p. 79).

- Pulsation in the posterior tibial artery (3) is normally palpable behind the medial malleolus (5), 2.5 cm in front of the medial border of the tendo calcaneus.

- The sustentaculum tali (12) is palpable about 2.5 cm below the tip of the medial malleolus (5).

Skeleton of the foot *bones of the left foot, from above*

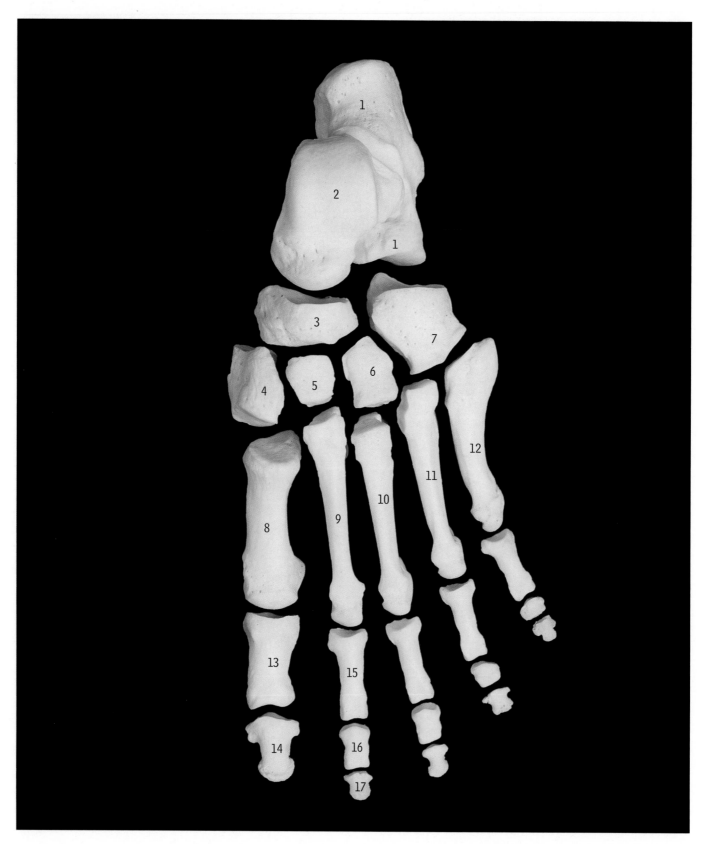

The talus and calcaneus remain articulated with each other but the remainder have been disarticulated.

1 Calcaneus
2 Talus
3 Navicular
4 Medial cuneiform
5 Intermediate cuneiform
6 Lateral cuneiform
7 Cuboid
8 First metatarsal
9 Second metatarsal
10 Third metatarsal
11 Fourth metatarsal
12 Fifth metatarsal
13 Proximal phalanx of great toe
14 Distal phalanx of great toe
15 Proximal phalanx of second toe
16 Middle phalanx of second toe
17 Distal phalanx of second toe

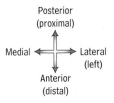

Posterior (proximal)

Medial ← → Lateral (left)

Anterior (distal)

- **Bones of the tarsus**
  Calcaneus
  Talus
  Navicular bone
  Cuboid bone
  Medial, intermediate and lateral cuneiform bones
- **Bones of the metatarsus**
  First to fifth metatarsal bones, numbered from medial to lateral
- **Bones of the toes or digits**
  Phalanges — a proximal and a distal phalanx for the great toe; proximal, middle and distal phalanges for each of the second to fifth toes
- The **hindfoot** consists of the talus and calcaneus.
- The **midfoot** consists of the navicular, cuboid and cuneiform bones.
- The **forefoot** consists of the metatarsal bones and phalanges.
- **Sesamoid bones** — two always present in the tendons of flexor hallucis brevis. For others see pp. 44, 46.
- **Origin and meaning of some names associated with the foot** are as follows (some older names for bones are given in parentheses):

Tibia:	Latin for a flute or pipe; when held upside down, the shin bone has a fanciful resemblance to this wind instrument.
Fibula:	Latin for a pin or skewer; the long thin bone of the leg. Adjective fibular or peroneal, which is from the Greek for pin (see the last note on p. 3).
Tarsus:	Greek for a wicker frame, in the basic framework for the back of the foot.
Metatarsus:	Greek for beyond the tarsus; the forepart of the foot.
Talus: (astragalus)	Latin (Greek) for one of a set of dice; viewed from above the main part of the talus has a rather square appearance.
Calcaneus: (os calcis, calcaneum)	From the Greek for heel; the heel bone.
Navicular: (scaphoid)	Latin (Greek) for boat-shaped; the navicular bone roughly resembles a saucer-shaped coracle.
Cuboid:	Greek for cube-shaped.
Cuneiform:	Latin for wedge-shaped.
Phalanx:	Greek for a row of soldiers; a row of bones in the toes. Plural phalanges.
Sesamoid:	Greek for shaped like a sesame seed.
Digitus:	Latin for finger or toe. Digiti and digitorum are the genitive singular and genitive plural — of the toe(s).
Hallux:	Latin for the great toe. Hallucis is the genitive singular — of the great toe.
Dorsum:	Latin for back; the upper surface of the foot. Adjective dorsal.
Plantar:	Adjective from planta, Latin for the sole of the foot.

Skeleton of the foot *articulated bones of the left foot*

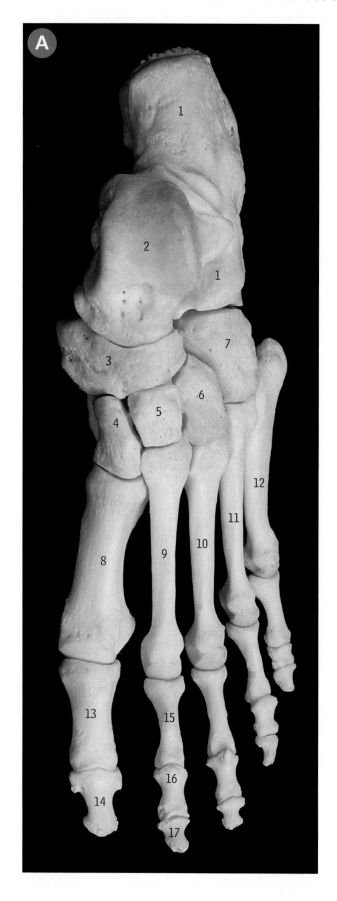

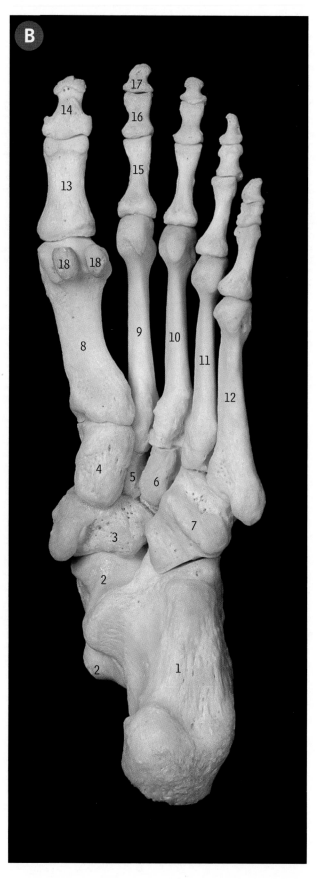

1 Calcaneus
2 Talus
3 Navicular
4 Medial cuneiform
5 Intermediate cuneiform
6 Lateral cuneiform
7 Cuboid
8 First metatarsal
9 Second metatarsal
10 Third metatarsal
11 Fourth metatarsal
12 Fifth metatarsal
13 Proximal phalanx of great toe
14 Distal phalanx of great toe
15 Proximal phalanx of second toe
16 Middle phalanx of second toe
17 Distal phalanx of second toe
18 Sesamoid bones

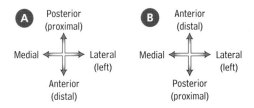

A from above (dorsal surface)

B from below (plantar surface)

Ossification of foot bones

All the tarsal bones are ossified from one primary center: calcaneus at the third fetal month, talus at the sixth fetal month, cuboid just before or just after birth, lateral cuneiform at 1 year, medial cuneiform at 2 years, intermediate cuneiform and navicular at 3 years.

The calcaneus is the only tarsal bone to have a secondary center: a thin plate of bone on the posterior surface, appearing at about 7 years and fusing during puberty.

The metatarsal bones and phalanges have primary centers for their shafts at the second to fourth fetal months, and one secondary center: at the base of the first metatarsal and bases of all the phalanges, but at the heads of the other metatarsals. These begin to ossify at 2 to 6 years and fuse at about 18 years.

All dates given are subject to considerable variation, and ossification tends to occur earlier in females.

- During the preparation of dried bones, the hyaline cartilage on articulating surfaces is lost, so that when rearticulating bones an exact fit is not possible. The thickness of the cartilage on joint surface is best appreciated in sections of bones, as on pp. 20, 21 and 92–104.

- The **talus** (2) is the uppermost foot bone, forming the ankle joint with the tibia and fibula. For details see pp. 52, 61.

- The **calcaneus** (1) is the most posterior and the largest foot bone, forming the heel. For details see pp. 62, 63.

- The **navicular bone** (3) lies in front of the talus, on the medial side of the foot. For details see p. 64.

- The **cuboid bone** (7) lies in front of the calcaneus, on the lateral side of the foot. For details see p. 64.

- The **three cuneiform bones** — medial, intermediate and lateral (4, 5 and 6) — lie in front of the navicular bone. For details see p. 65.

- The first, second and third **metatarsal bones** (8, 9 and 10) are in front of the three cuneiforms, and the fourth and fifth metatarsal bones (11 and 12) are in front of the cuboid bone. For details see pp. 66, 67.

- The **phalanges** (13–17) are the bones of the toes. Each proximal phalanx articulates with the head of a metatarsal bone. Each phalanx has a base (at the proximal end), body and head (at the distal end). The body is convex on the dorsal (upper) surface, and concave on the plantar surface. See pp. 42, 50.

Skeleton of the foot
Attachments of muscles and major ligaments to the bones of the left foot

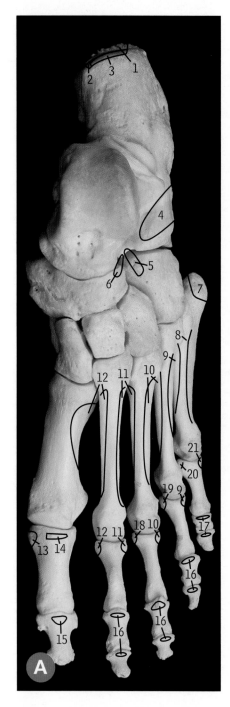

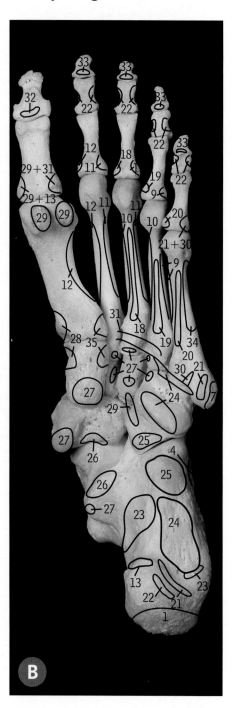

1   Tendo calcaneus
2   Plantaris
3   Area for bursa
4   Extensor digitorum brevis
5   Calcaneocuboid part   } of bifurcate
6   Calcaneonavicular part   ligament
7   Fibularis (*peroneus*) brevis
8   Fibularis (*peroneus*) tertius
9   Fourth
10 Third   } dorsal interosseus
11 Second
12 First
13 Abductor hallucis
14 Extensor hallucis brevis
15 Extensor hallucis longus
16 Extensor digitorum longus and brevis
17 Extensor digitorum longus
18 First
19 Second   } plantar interosseus
20 Third
21 Abductor digiti minimi
22 Flexor digitorum brevis
23 Quadratus plantae
24 Long plantar ligament
25 Plantar calcaneocuboid (short plantar) ligament
26 Plantar calcaneonavicular (spring) ligament
27 Tibialis posterior
28 Tibialis anterior
29 Flexor hallucis brevis
30 Flexor digiti minimi brevis
31 Adductor hallucis
32 Flexor hallucis longus
33 Flexor digitorum longus
34 Opponens digiti minimi (occasional part of **30**)
35 Fibularis (*peroneus*) longus

A from above (dorsal surface)

B from below (plantar surface)

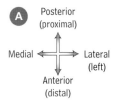

A   Posterior (proximal)

Medial ← → Lateral (left)

Anterior (distal)

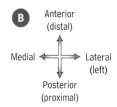

B   Anterior (distal)

Medial ← → Lateral (left)

Posterior (proximal)

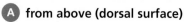

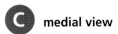

Sesamoid and Accessory bones

Sesamoid bones

The patella is by far the largest sesamoid bone in the lower limb and its close association with tendons and a bony joint (the knee), gives a conceptual focus as to the function of sesamoid bones.

In the Foot:

- They usually vary in shape and size but in general are ovoid and normally only a few millimeters in diameter (p. 44, **B18**).

- They are not always ossified but may consist of fibrous tissue or cartilage, or a combination of all three.

- They are usually found embedded in tendons at the point where the tendons angle acutely around bony surfaces to their point of insertion (p. 92, **16** and p. 93, **33**.

- Sesamoids have articular cartilage on the surface which is in direct relationship to the bone that they are proximate too.

Although not proved, it is thought that sesamoid bones protect tendons from wear, and by their strategic position to joints, alter the angle of insertion of a tendon into bone and thus provides a greater mechanical advantage to the joint.

Accessory bones

Bones within the human body gradually begin to form during the early developmental phases of the fetus by the initial formation of central areas of ossification within the cartilaginous and membranous skeleton. These ossified areas continue to grow, unite and eventually form solid adult bones, some during late childhood and some as late as early adulthood.

On occasions however the centres of ossification fail to fuse completely, often at the ends of bones, and thus a separate (accessory or supernumerary) bone is formed.

The foot is a common place for accessory bones to form and there are common sites for them to occur. It is important to be aware of their possible presence because on a radiographic image they can be easily mistaken for a fractured bone or 'chip'.

Common accessory bones in the foot are:

- **Dorsum of foot**
  Os intercuneiforme
  Os talonaviculare dorsale
  Os calcaneus secondarius
  Os intermetatarsal I

- **Posterior part of foot**
  Os trigonum

- **Lateral part of foot**
  Os calcaneus secondarius
  Os vesalianum pedis

- **Medial part of foot**
  Os tibiale externum (Os naviculare accessorium)
  Os sustentaculi

- **Plantar aspect (sole) of foot**
  Pars peronea metatarsalis I
  Os cuboides secondarius

C   medial view

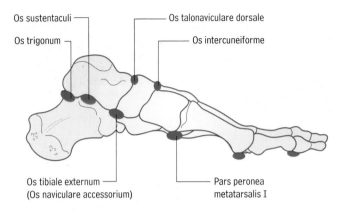

Os sustentaculi —   Os talonaviculare dorsale
Os trigonum   Os intercuneiforme
Os tibiale externum —   Pars peronea
(Os naviculare accessorium)   metatarsalis I

D   lateral view

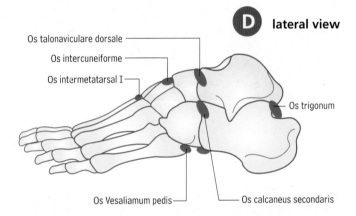

Os talonaviculare dorsale —
Os intercuneiforme —
Os intermetatarsal I —
Os trigonum
Os Vesaliamum pedis —   Os calcaneus secondaris

E

inferior (plantar) view

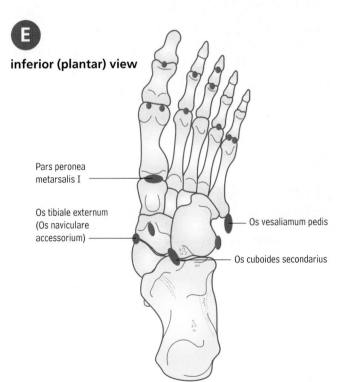

Pars peronea metarsalis I —
Os tibiale externum (Os naviculare accessorium) —
Os vesaliamum pedis
Os cuboides secondarius

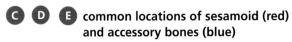

C   **D**   **E**   common locations of sesamoid (red) and accessory bones (blue)

Skeleton of the foot
Articulated bones of the left foot

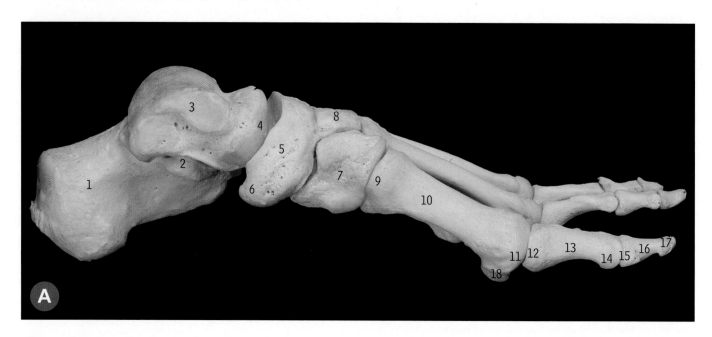

A from the medial side

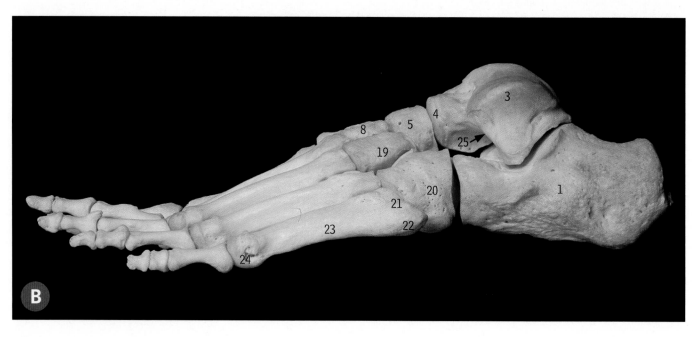

B from the lateral side

1 Body of calcaneus
2 Sustentaculum tali part of calcaneus
3 Body of talus
4 Head of talus
5 Navicular
6 Tuberosity of navicular
7 Medial cuneiform
8 Intermediate cuneiform
9 Base ⎫
10 Body ⎬ of first metatarsal
11 Head ⎭
12 Base ⎫
13 Body ⎬ of proximal phalanx of great toe
14 Head ⎭
15 Base ⎫
16 Body ⎬ of distal phalanx of great toe
17 Head ⎭
18 Sesamoid bone
19 Lateral cuneiform
20 Cuboid
21 Base ⎫
22 Tuberosity ⎬ of fifth metatarsal
23 Body ⎪
24 Head ⎭
25 Tarsal sinus

- When standing (as can be seen from the imprint of a wet foot on the floor or when viewed through a glass plate — see p. 39, **F**) the parts of the foot in contact with the ground are the heel, the lateral margin of the foot, the pads under the metatarsal heads and the pads under the distal part of the toes.

- The medial margin of the foot is not normally in contact with the ground because of the height of the medial longitudinal arch (see pp. 50 and 51). In flat foot the medial arch is lower with an increasingly large imprint on the medial side.

- The body weight when standing is borne by the tuberosity of the calcaneus and the heads of the metatarsals, especially the first (with the sesamoid bones underneath it) and the fifth. As the foot bends forward in walking the other metatarsal heads take increasingly more of the load. With further raising of the heel the toe pads become pressed to the ground and so take some of the weight off the metatarsals.

- Although the forearm and hand have many muscles similar in name and action to those of the leg and foot, their normal use in everyday life is different. In the upper limb the muscles work from above to produce intricate movements of the thumb and fingers in a free limb.
  In the lower limb the toes must be stabilized on the ground so that muscles can work from below to produce the propulsive movements of walking.

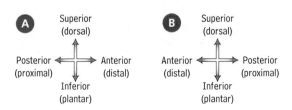

Skeleton of the foot
Bones of the left longitudinal arches, transverse tarsal joint and other joints

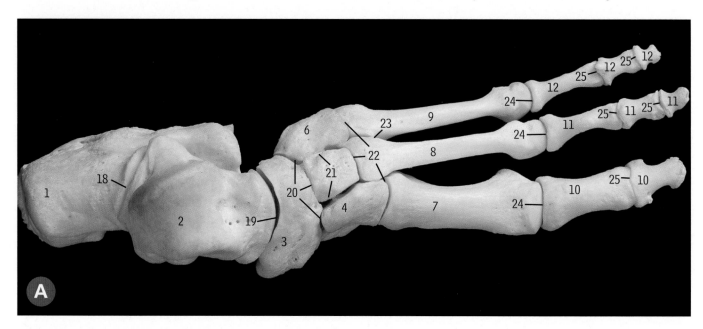

A bones of the medial longitudinal arch, from above

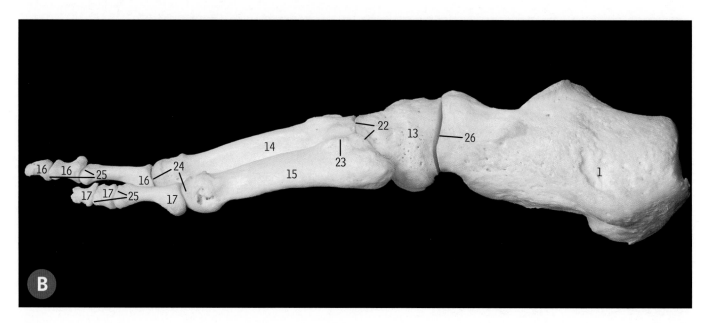

B bones of the lateral longitudinal arch, from the lateral side

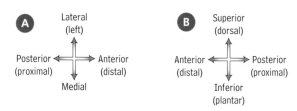

A
Lateral
(left)

Posterior ⟷ Anterior
(proximal)   (distal)

Medial

B
Superior
(dorsal)

Anterior ⟷ Posterior
(distal)   (proximal)

Inferior
(plantar)

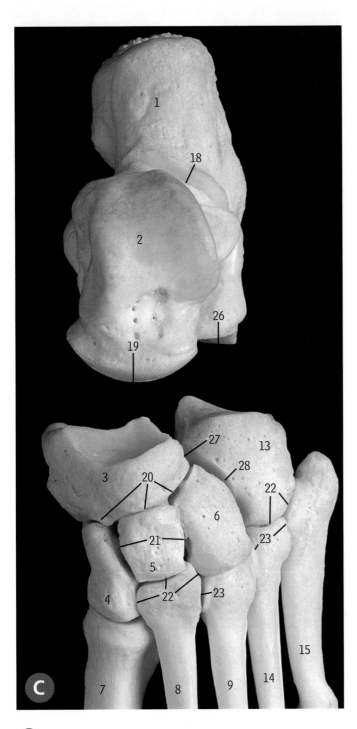

- The bones of the medial longitudinal arch (**A**) are the calcaneus, talus, navicular, the three cuneiforms and the medial three metatarsal bones.
- The bones of the lateral longitudinal arch (**B**) are the calcaneus, cuboid and the two lateral metatarsal bones.
- The transverse arch is formed by the cuboid and cuneiform bones and the adjacent parts of the five metatarsals (those of each foot forming one half of the whole arch). At the level of the metatarsal heads the arched form is no longer present.
- The medial longitudinal arch is higher than the lateral.
- While the shape of the individual bones determines the shapes of the arches, the *maintenance* of the arches in the *stationary* foot (standing in the normal upright position) depends largely on the ligaments in the sole (where they are larger and stronger than those on the dorsum). As soon as movement occurs the long tendons and small muscles of the sole assume importance in maintaining the curved forms.
- The many joints of the foot contribute to its function as a *flexible* lever, and the word arch suggests an architectural rigidity that does not exist.
- On the medial side the plantar calcaneonavicular ligament (spring ligament) is of particular importance in supporting the head of the talus, and other structures that help to maintain the medial arch include the plantar aponeurosis, flexor hallucis longus, tibialis anterior and posterior, and the medial parts of flexor digitorum longus and brevis.
- The transverse tarsal joint (midtarsal joint) is the collective name for two joints — the calcaneocuboid joint, and the talonavicular part of the talocalcaneonavicular joint.

C the transverse tarsal joint, disarticulated, from above

C
Posterior (proximal)
Medial ⟷ Lateral (left)
Anterior (distal)

1   Calcaneus
2   Talus
3   Navicular
4   Medial cuneiform
5   Intermediate cuneiform
6   Lateral cuneiform
7   First metatarsal
8   Second metatarsal
9   Third metatarsal
10 Phalanges of great toe
11 Phalanges of second toe
12 Phalanges of third toe
13 Cuboid
14 Fourth metatarsal
15 Fifth metatarsal
16 Phalanges of fourth toe
17 Phalanges of fifth toe
18 Talocalcanean joint
19 Talonavicular part of talocalcaneonavicular joint
20 Cuneonavicular joint
21 Intercuneiform joints
22 Tarsometatarsal joints (cuneometatarsal and cuboideometatarsal)
23 Intermetatarsal joints
24 Metatarsophalangeal joints
25 Interphalangeal joints
26 Calcaneocuboid joint
27 Cuboideonavicular joint
28 Cuneocuboid joint

Foot bones *left talus*

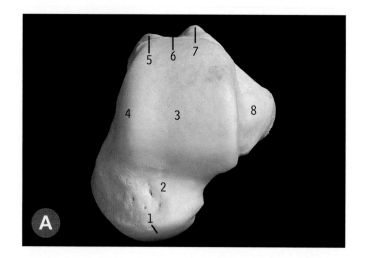

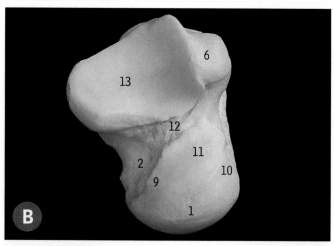

A **from above**

Posterior
(proximal)

Medial ◄────► Lateral
(left)

Anterior
(distal)

B **from below**

Posterior
(proximal)

Lateral ◄────► Medial
(left)

Anterior
(distal)

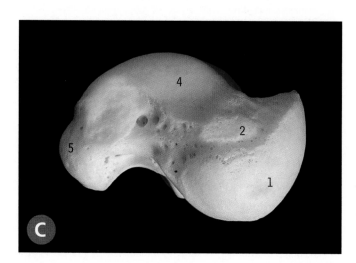

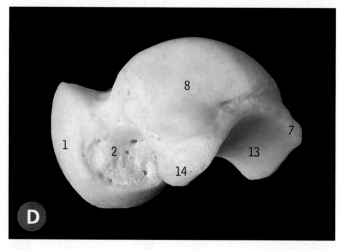

C **from the medial side**

Superior
(dorsal)

Posterior ◄────► Anterior
(proximal)   (distal)

Inferior
(plantar)

D **from the lateral side**

Superior
(dorsal)

Anterior ◄────► Posterior
(distal)   (proximal)

Inferior
(plantar)

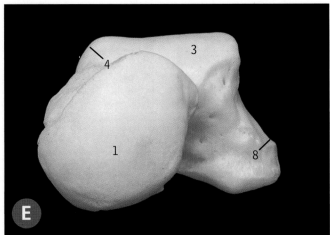

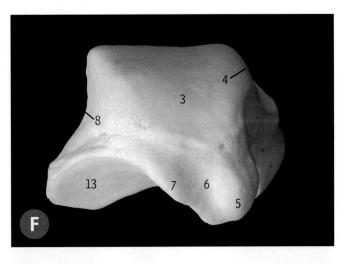

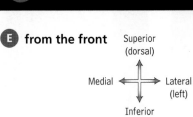

E **from the front**

Superior
(dorsal)

Medial ⟷ Lateral
(left)

Inferior
(plantar)

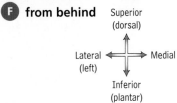

F **from behind**

Superior
(dorsal)

Lateral ⟷ Medial
(left)

Inferior
(plantar)

1 Head with articular surface for navicular
2 Neck
3 Trochlear surface of body, for inferior surface of tibia
4 Surface for medial malleolus
5 Medial tubercle
6 Groove for flexor hallucis longus tendon ⎫ of posterior process
7 Lateral tubercle ⎬
8 Surface for lateral malleolus ⎭
9 Anterior calcanean articular surface
10 Surface for plantar calcaneonavicular (spring) ligament
11 Middle calcanean articular surface
12 Sulcus tali
13 Posterior calcanean articular surface
14 Lateral process

Talus

• The uppermost foot bone, forming the ankle joint with the tibia and fibula.

• Formerly known as the astragalus.

• Articular facets on the upper surface and sides for the tibia and fibula, on the under surface for the calcaneus, and on the anterior surface (head) for the navicular.

• Unique among the foot bones in having no muscles attached to it.

Foot bones *left talus and the lower ends of the tibia and fibula*

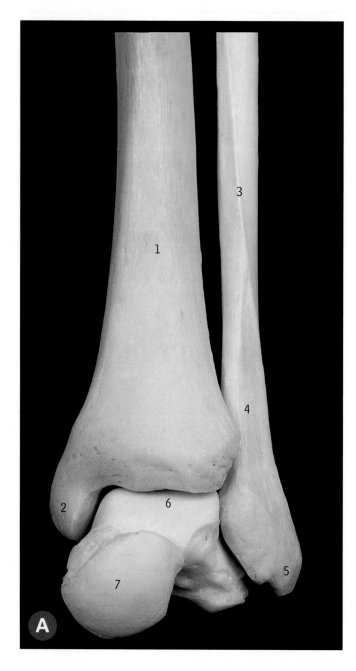

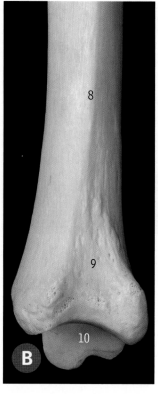

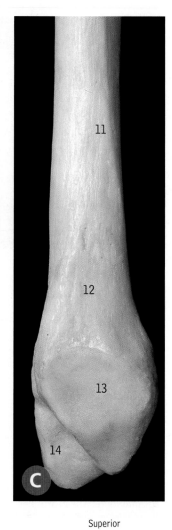

Superior
(proximal)

Anterior ←→ Posterior

Inferior
(distal)

Superior
(proximal)

Posterior ←→ Anterior

Inferior
(distal)

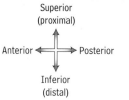

A the talus, tibia and fibula,
articulated, from the front

B the tibia from the lateral side

C the fibula from the medial side

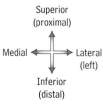

Superior
(proximal)

Medial ←→ Lateral
(left)

Inferior
(distal)

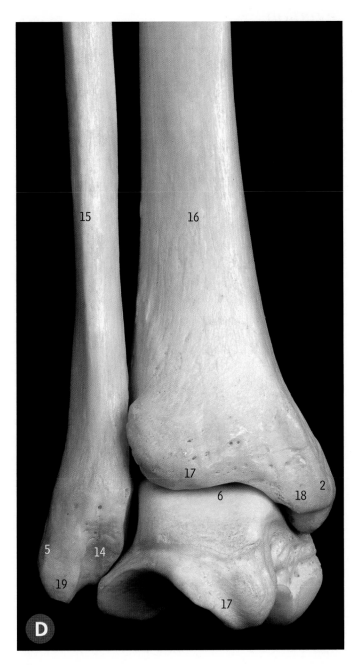

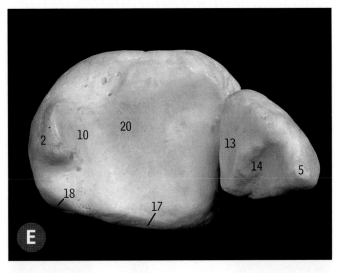

E the tibia and fibula, articulated, from below

Anterior

Medial ←→ Lateral
(left)

Posterior

1	Anterior surface ⎫ of tibia
2	Medial malleolus ⎭
3	Anterior border ⎫
4	Triangular subcutaneous area ⎬ of fibula
5	Lateral malleolus ⎭
6	Trochlear surface of body ⎫ of talus
7	Head ⎭
8	Interosseous border ⎫
9	Fibular notch ⎬ of tibia
10	Articular (lateral) surface of medial malleolus ⎭
11	Interosseous border ⎫
12	Surface for interosseous tibiofibularis ligament ⎪
13	Articular (medial) surface of lateral malleolus ⎬ of fibula
14	Malleolar fossa ⎪
15	Posterior border ⎭
16	Posterior surface of tibia
17	Groove for flexor hallucis longus tendon
18	Groove for tibialis posterior tendon
19	Groove for fibularis (*peroneus*) brevis tendon
20	Inferior surface of tibia

D the talus, tibia and fibula, articulated, from behind

Superior
(proximal)

Lateral ←→ Medial
(left)

Inferior
(distal)

Foot bones *left talus and the lower ends of the tibia and fibula, with ligamentous attachments in the ankle region*

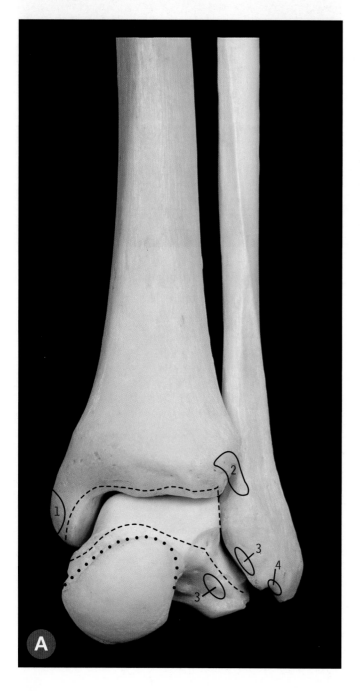

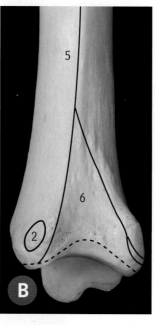

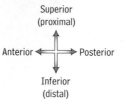

Superior
(proximal)

Anterior ←→ Posterior

Inferior
(distal)

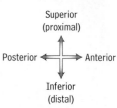

B the tibia from the lateral side
C the fibula from the medial side

Superior
(proximal)

Posterior ←→ Anterior

Inferior
(distal)

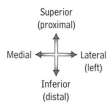

A the talus, tibia and fibula, articulated, from the front

Superior
(proximal)

Medial ←→ Lateral
(left)

Inferior
(distal)

The attachment of the capsule of the ankle joint is indicated by the dashed line, and that of the talocalcaneonavicular joint by the dotted line.

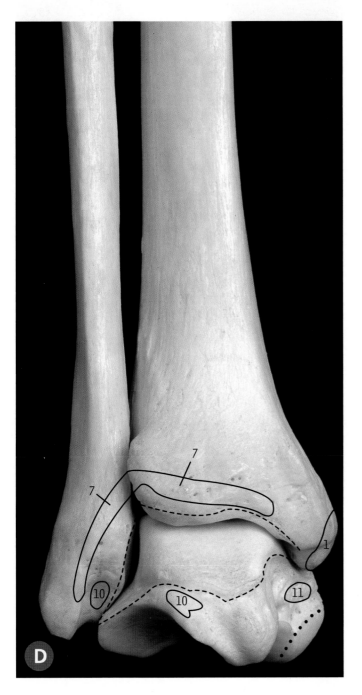

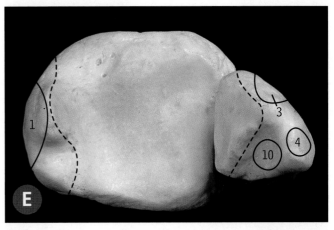

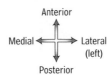

E the tibia and fibula, articulated, from below

Anterior

Medial ⟷ Lateral (left)

Posterior

1 Medial (deltoid) ligament
2 Anterior tibiofibular ligament
3 Anterior talofibular ligament
4 Calcaneofibular ligament
5 Interosseous membrane
6 Interosseous tibiofibular ligament
7 Posterior tibiofibular ligament
8 Fibularis (*peroneus*) tertius
9 Flexor hallucis longus
10 Posterior talofibular ligament
11 Deep part of medial (deltoid) ligament

• The interosseous tibiofibular ligament (**B** and **C, 6**) is the main bond of union of the inferior tibiofibular joint.

D the talus, tibia and fibula, articulated, from behind

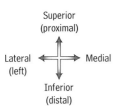

Superior (proximal)

Lateral (left) ⟷ Medial

Inferior (distal)

Foot bones *left talus and the lower ends of the tibia and fibula*

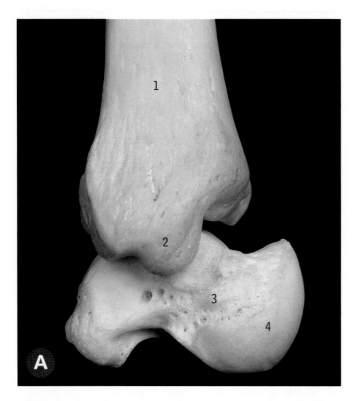

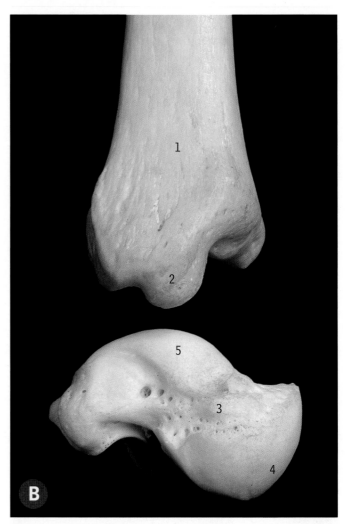

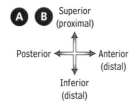

A the talus and tibia, articulated, from the medial side

A **B** Superior (proximal)

Posterior ← → Anterior (distal)

Inferior (distal)

B the talus and tibia, disarticulated, from the medial side

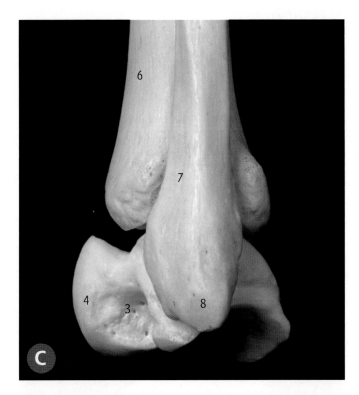

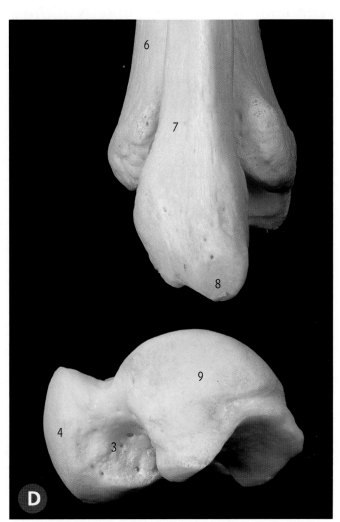

C the talus, tibia and fibula, articulated, from the lateral side

1 Medial surface ⎫ of tibia
2 Medial malleolus ⎭
3 Neck ⎫ of talus
4 Head ⎭
5 Surface for medial malleolus
6 Anterior surface of tibia
7 Triangular subcutaneous surface ⎫ of fibula
8 Lateral malleolus ⎭
9 Surface for lateral malleolus

D the talus disarticulated from the tibia and fibula, from the lateral side

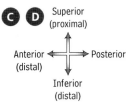

C **D** Superior (proximal)

Anterior (distal) ← → Posterior

Inferior (distal)

Foot bones *left talus and the lower ends of the tibia and fibula, with ligamentous attachments in the ankle region*

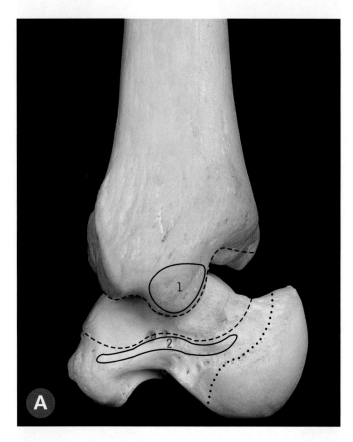

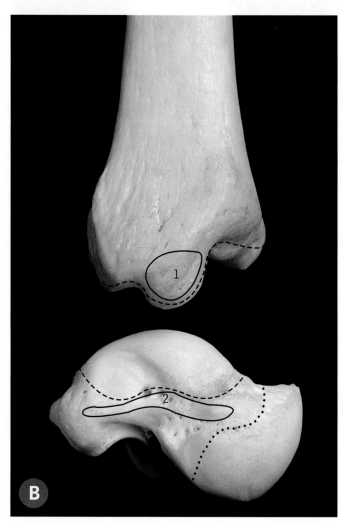

A   the talus and tibia, articulated, from the medial side

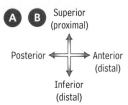

A **B**   Superior (proximal)

Posterior ⟷ Anterior (distal)

Inferior (distal)

B   the talus and tibia, disarticulated, from the medial side

The attachment of the capsule of the ankle joint is indicated by the
dashed line, and that of the talocalcaneonavicular joint by the dotted line.

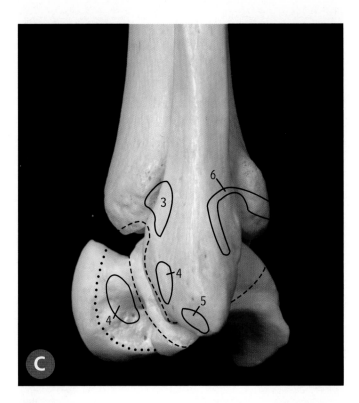

C the talus, tibia and fibula, articulated, from the
lateral side

1 Medial (deltoid) ligament
2 Deep part of medial (deltoid) ligament
3 Anterior tibiofibular ligament
4 Anterior talofibular ligament
5 Calcaneofibular ligament
6 Posterior tibiofibular ligament

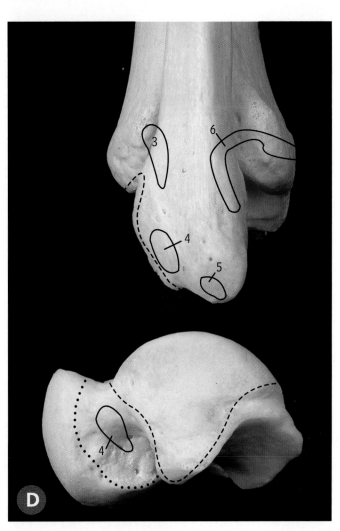

D the talus disarticulated from the tibia and fibula,
from the lateral side

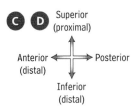

C **D** Superior
(proximal)

Anterior ← → Posterior
(distal)

Inferior
(distal)

Foot bones *left calcaneus*

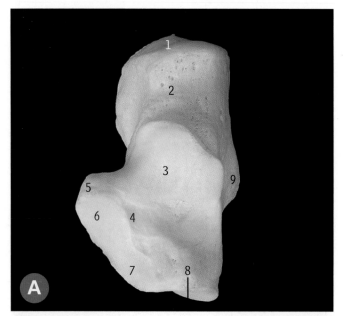

A from above

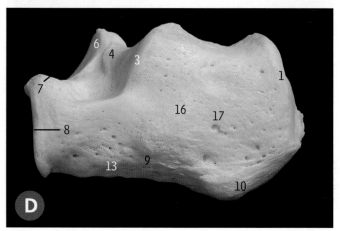

B from below

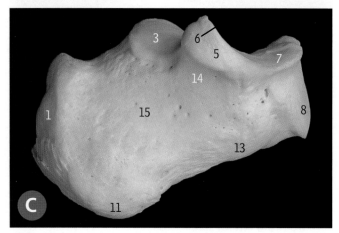

C from the medial side

D from the lateral side

1 Posterior surface
2 Dorsal surface
3 Posterior articular surface for talus
4 Sulcus calcanei
5 Sustentaculum tali
6 Middle articular surface for talus
7 Anterior articular surface for talus
8 Articular surface for cuboid
9 Fibular (*peroneal*) trochlea
10 Lateral process ⎫
11 Medial process ⎬ of tuberosity
12 Plantar surface
13 Anterior tubercle
14 Groove for flexor hallucis longus tendon
15 Medial surface

16 Lateral surface
17 Tubercle for calcaneofibular ligament
18 Surface for bursa
19 Surface for tendo calcaneus
20 Surface for fibrofatty tissue
21 Medial ⎫
22 Lateral ⎬ talocalcanean ligament
23 Tibiocalcanean part of medial (deltoid) ligament
24 Interosseous talocalcanean ligament
25 Inferior extensor retinaculum
26 Cervical ligament
27 Extensor digitorum brevis
28 Calcaneocuboid part
29 Calcaneonavicular part of bifurcate ligament

The capsule of the talocalcanean joint is indicated by the dashed line, and that of the talocalcanean part of the talocalcaneonavicular joint by the dotted line.

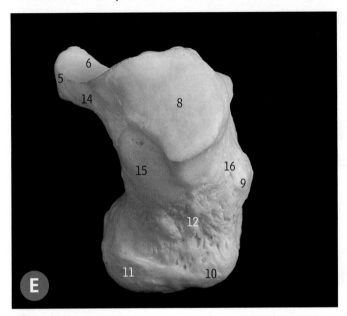

E from the front

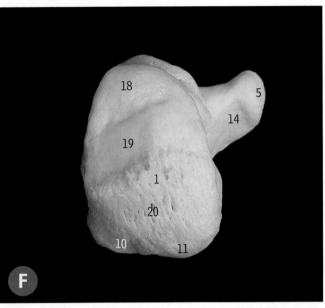

F from behind

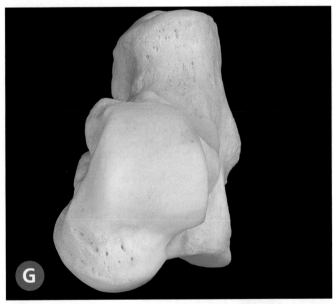

G articulated with the talus, from above

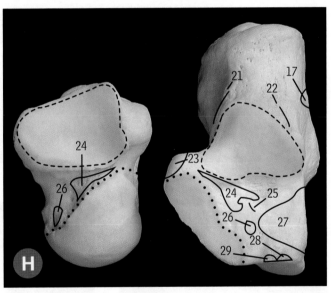

H with the talus disarticulated and turned upside down, with attachments

Calcaneus

- The largest foot bone, forming the heel.
- Formerly known as the calcaneum or os calcis.
- Articular facets on the upper surface for the talus and on the anterior surface for the cuboid.
- Prominent sustentaculum tali projecting medially.
- When the talus and calcaneus are articulated the sulcus tali (see p. 52, **B12**) and sulcus calcanei (4) form the tarsal sinus (sinus tarsi).

Foot bones

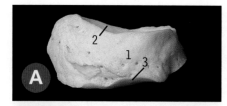

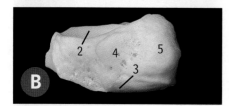

A from above

B from below

C proximal aspect

D distal aspect

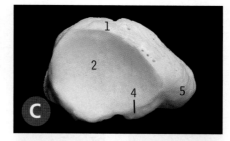

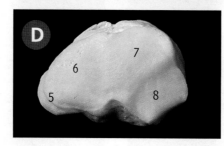

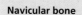

Left navicular bone

1 Dorsal surface
2 Proximal surface for talus
3 Distal surface for cuneiforms
4 Plantar surface
5 Tuberosity
6 Facet for medial cuneiform
7 Facet for intermediate cuneiform } on distal surface
8 Facet for lateral cuneiform

Navicular bone

• Formerly known as the scaphoid bone.

• Posterior articular facet for the talus; anterior articular facet for the three cuneiforms.

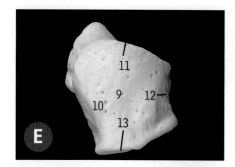

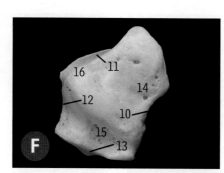

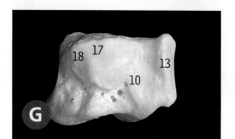

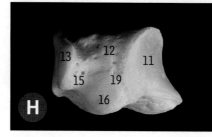

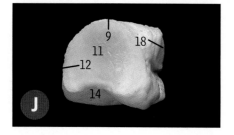

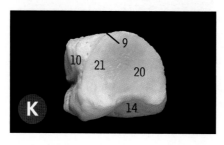

Left cuboid bone

E from above

F from below

G from the medial side

H from the lateral side

J proximal aspect

K distal aspect

9 Dorsal surface
10 Medial surface
11 Proximal surface for calcaneus
12 Lateral surface
13 Distal surface
14 Plantar surface
15 Groove for fibularis (peroneus) longus tendon
16 Tuberosity
17 Surface for lateral cuneiform
18 Surface for navicular
19 Facet for sesamoid bone in fibularis (peroneus) longus tendon
20 Facet for fifth metatarsal } on distal
21 Facet for fourth metatarsal } surface

Cuboid bone

• Posterior articular facet for the calcaneus; anterior articular facet for the fourth and fifth metatarsals.

• Groove on the under surface for the tendon of fibularis (peroneus) longus.

Articulated left cuneiform bones (medial, intermediate and lateral)

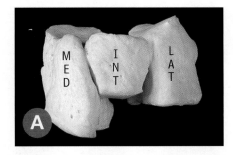

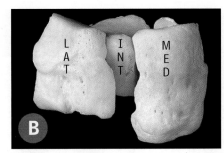

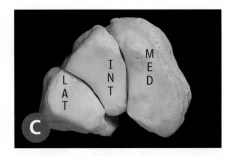

(A) **from above**

(B) **from below**

(C) **proximal (navicular) aspect (for distal aspect see p. 66)**

Left medial cuneiform bone

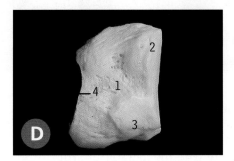

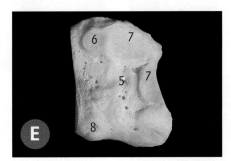

(D) **from the medial side**

(E) **from the lateral side**

> **Cuneiform bones**
> - Medial (the largest), intermediate (the smallest), and lateral.
> - Situated between the navicular and the first three metatarsals.

1 Medial surface
2 Distal surface for first metatarsal
3 Area for tendon of tibialis anterior
4 Proximal surface for navicular
5 Lateral surface
6 Surface for second metatarsal
7 Surface for intermediate cuneiform
8 Area for fibularis (*peroneus*) longus tendon
9 Medial surface
10 Surface for medial cuneiform
11 Distal surface for second metatarsal
12 Lateral surface
13 Surface for lateral cuneiform
14 Proximal surface for navicular
15 Medial surface
16 Surfaces for second metatarsal
17 Surface for intermediate cuneiform
18 Proximal surface for navicular
19 Lateral surface
20 Surface for cuboid
21 Surface for fourth metatarsal
22 Distal surface for third metatarsal

Left intermediate cuneiform bone

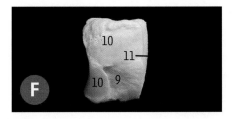

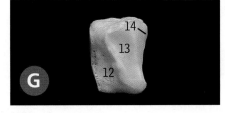

(F) **from the medial side**

(G) **from the lateral side**

Left lateral cuneiform bone

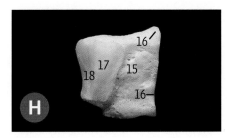

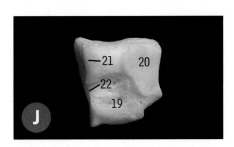

(H) **from the medial side**

(J) **from the lateral side**

Foot bones

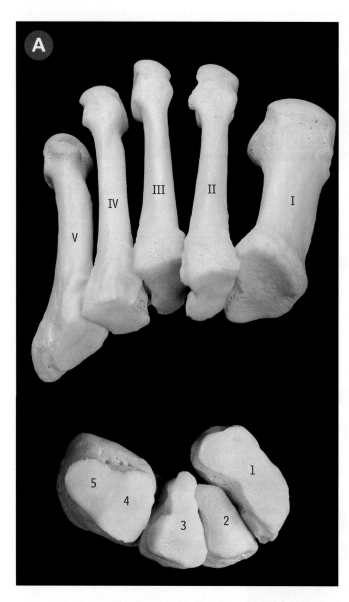

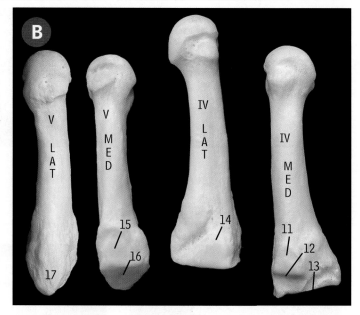

The metatarsal bones are articulated with each other but have been disarticulated from the cuneiform and cuboid bones, which have been rotated to show the surfaces that articulate with the metatarsals. For orientation see articulated foot (p. 44).

1   Surface of medial cuneiform for first metatarsal
2   Surface of intermediate cuneiform for second metatarsal
3   Surface of lateral cuneiform for third metatarsal
4   Surface of cuboid for fourth metatarsal
5   Surface of cuboid for fifth metatarsal

The base of the third metatarsal articulates with the lateral cuneiform and the bases of the second and fourth metatarsals.

The base of the fourth metatarsal articulates with the lateral cuneiform and the cuboid and the base of the fifth metatarsal.

The base of the fifth metatarsal articulates with the cuboid and the base of the fourth metatarsal

A left cuneiform, cuboid and metatarsal bones articulated, from above and in front

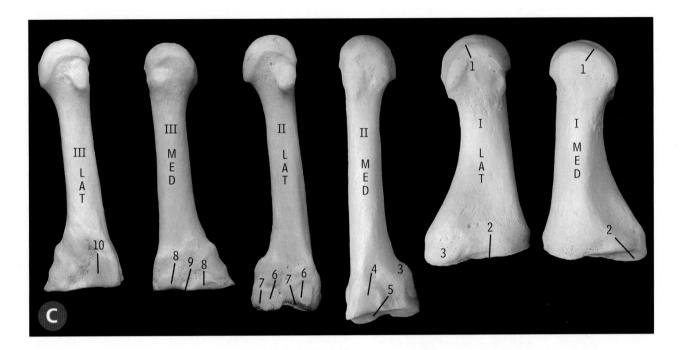

B **C** left metatarsal bones—numbered I–V with their medial and lateral sides named

The bones are arranged on their sides so that the articular surfaces on the adjacent sides of their bases can be seen, for orientation see articulated foot (p. 44).

1 Groove on head for sesamoid bone
2 Surface for medial cuneiform
3 Area for bursa
4 Surface for medial cuneiform
5 Surface for intermediate cuneiform
6 Surfaces for third metatarsal
7 Surfaces for lateral cuneiform
8 Surfaces for second metatarsal
9 Surface for lateral cuneiform
10 Surface for fourth metatarsal
11 Surface for third metatarsal
12 Surface for lateral cuneiform
13 Surface for cuboid
14 Surface for fifth metatarsal
15 Surface for fourth metatarsal
16 Surface for cuboid
17 Tuberosity of base

Metatarsal bones

- First to fifth, leading to each toe and each with a base (at the proximal or ankle end), body or shaft, and head (at the toe end). Bases of first three articulate with cuneiform bones; bases of fourth and fifth articulate with the cuboid. Heads articulate with bases of proximal phalanges.

- The second, third and fourth metatarsals are longer than the first and fifth; the first is the shortest and the thickest.

- The second metatarsal is the longest bone and its base is recessed between the medial and lateral cuneiforms as well as articulating with the intermediate cuneiform (forming a Keystone). Thus, the second metatarsal is the most rigid of the metatarsals.

- The cuneiforms and bases of the metatarsals are wedge shaped to help form a bony arch.

- Refer to an articulated foot (p. 44) and note the following:

  The base of the first metatarsal articulates with the medial cuneiform. There is normally a bursa but not a joint between the bases of the first and second metatarsals.

  The base of the second metatarsal articulates with all three cuneiforms and with the base of the third metatarsal. This second metatarsal base extends more proximally than the first and third bases—an interlocking device that prevents side-to-side movement.

Lower leg and foot

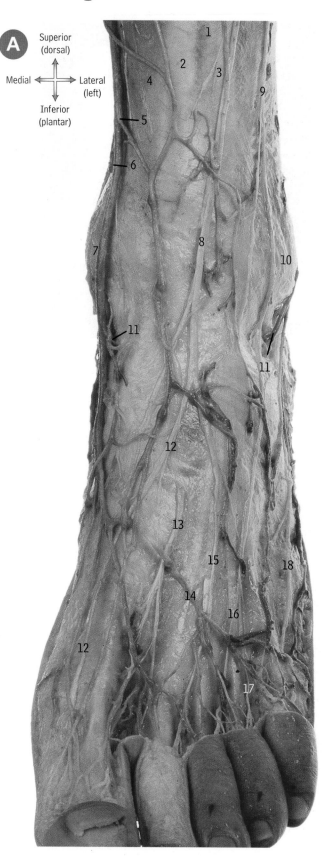

A Superior (dorsal)

Medial ← → Lateral (left)

Inferior (plantar)

A superficial vessels and nerves of the left lower leg and foot, from the front

Skin and superficial connective tissue have been removed to show the superficial vessels and nerves lying on the deep fascia (**1**). In **A** the medial side of the dorsal venous arch (**14**) joins the medial marginal vein of the foot to form the great saphenous vein (**5**), which runs up in front of the medial malleolus (**7**). The medial and lateral branches of the superficial fibular (*peroneal*) nerve (**8** and **9**) pass down on to the dorsum, supplemented on the medial side by the saphenous nerve (**6**) and on the lateral side by the sural nerve (**18**). The end of the deep fibular (*peroneal*) nerve (**13**) perforates the deep fascia to run to the first toe cleft.

1 Deep fascia
2 Tendon of tibialis anterior (under fascia)
3 Tendon of extensor digitorum longus (under fascia)
4 Medial surface of tibia (under fascia)
5 Great saphenous vein
6 Saphenous nerve
7 Medial malleolus
8 Medial branch of superficial fibular (*peroneal*) nerve
9 Lateral branch of superficial fibular (*peroneal*) nerve
10 Lateral malleolus
11 A perforating vein
12 Proper dorsal digital nerve of great toe
13 Medial terminal branch of deep fibular (*peroneal*) nerve
14 Dorsal venous arch
15 Dorsal digital nerve to second cleft
16 Dorsal digital nerve to third cleft
17 Dorsal digital nerve to fourth cleft
18 Sural nerve

- The skin of the first toe cleft is supplied by the *deep* fibular (peroneal) nerve (**A13**); the skin of the other clefts is supplied by the *superficial* fibular (peroneal) nerve (**A8** and **9**).

- The skin behind the ankle and at the back of the heel is supplied on the medial side by the saphenous nerve (**A6**, from the femoral nerve) and the medial calcanean branches (**B8**) of the tibial nerve, and on the lateral side by the sural nerve (**B2**, also from the tibial nerve).

- The saphenous nerve (**A6**) on the medial side of the foot supplies skin as far forward as the metatarsophalangeal joint of the great toe.

- The sural nerve (**A18**) on the lateral side of the foot supplies skin as far forward as the side of the fifth toe.

- The skin of the medial side of the dorsum of the foot, including the region of the medial malleolus, is part of the fourth lumbar dermatome (**Fig. 9**, p. 121). The fifth lumbar dermatome includes the rest of the dorsum, and the first sacral dermatome includes the lateral side of the foot and the lateral malleolar region.

- The *great* saphenous vein (**A5**) passes upward in front of the *medial* malleolus (**A7**).

- The *small* saphenous vein (**B3**) passes upward behind the *lateral* malleolus (**B11**).

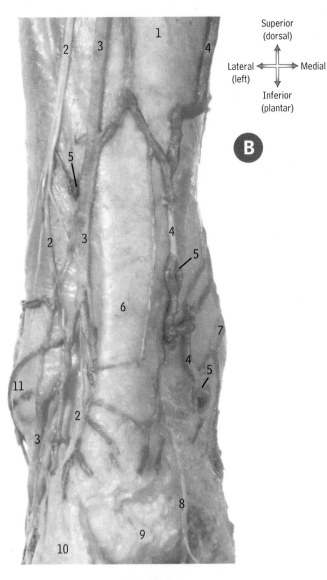

Superior
(dorsal)

Lateral ←→ Medial
(left)

Inferior
(plantar)

B

B superficial vessels and nerves of the left lower leg and foot, from behind

In B the most obvious structure is the tendo calcaneus (Achilles' tendon, 6), running down to be attached to the back of the calcaneus (9). The small saphenous vein (3) and sural nerve (2) with their tributaries and branches are behind the lateral malleous (11). On both sides but especially the medial, there are some typical perforating veins (5), piercing the deep fascia to form communications between the superficial and deep veins. The posterior arch vein (4) unites several of the perforators on the medial side.

1 Deep fascia
2 Sural nerve
3 Small saphenous vein
4 Posterior arch vein
5 A perforating vein
6 Tendo calcaneus (under fascia)
7 Medial malleolus
8 Medial calcanean nerve
9 Posterior surface of calcaneus
10 Fibrofatty tissue of heel
11 Lateral malleolus

C axial cross section of the left leg above the level of the upper part of B

The section in C is viewed from below, looking from the ankle toward the knee. Tibialis posterior (13) is the deepest of the calf muscles (immediately behind the interosseous membrane, 5) with the tibial nerve (19) behind it and the posterior tibial vessels (20) more medially, between flexor digitorum longus (21) and soleus (14). The fibular (*peroneal*) artery (12) is adjacent to flexor hallucis longus (11) behind the fibula (8). Note the (unlabeled) dilated veins within and deep to soleus (14); they are the site for potentially dangerous deep venous thrombosis. In the anterior compartment, in front of the interosseous membrane (5), the anterior tibial vessels (3) and deep fibular (*peroneal*) nerve (4) are between tibialis anterior (2) and extensor hallucis longus (6).

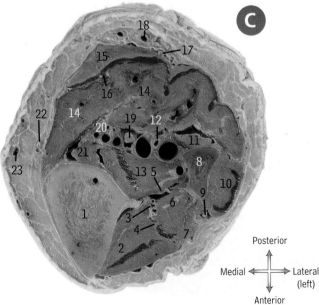

C

Posterior

Medial ←→ Lateral
(left)

Anterior

1 Tibia	11 Flexor hallucis longus
2 Tibialis anterior	12 Fibular (*peroneal*) artery
3 Anterior tibial vessels	13 Tibialis posterior
4 Deep fibular (*peroneal*) nerve	14 Soleus
5 Interosseous membrane	15 Gastrocnemius
6 Extensor hallucis longus	16 Plantaris tendon
7 Extensor digitorum longus	17 Sural nerve
8 Fibula	18 Small saphenous vein
9 Superficial fibular (*peroneal*) nerve	19 Tibial nerve
10 Fibularis (*peroneus*) longus and brevis	20 Posterior tibial vessels
	21 Flexor digitorum longus
	22 Saphenous nerve
	23 Great saphenous vein

Lower leg and foot

This medial view emphasizes the position of the great saphenous vein (3) in front of the medial malleolus (5), with branches of the saphenous nerve (4) lying both in front of and behind the vein. There are perforating veins (9) behind the malleolus and joining the posterior arch vein (12), and a large medial calcanean branch (10) of the tibial nerve running down to the skin of the heel.

- In the specimen shown on pp. 68–71 some of the superficial veins are rather dilated and tortuous, but this has served to emphasize the posterior arch vein and perforating veins.

- The perforating veins (**A9, B8**) serve as communications between the superficial veins (above the deep fascia) and deep veins (below the fascia). Many of these communicating vessels possess valves that direct the flow of blood from superficial to deep; venous return from the limb is then brought about by the pumping action of the muscles (which are all below the deep fascia). If the valves become incompetent or the deep veins are blocked, pressure in the superficial veins increases and they become varicose (from the Latin for an enlarged and tortuous vessel).

- Perforating veins are variable in number and position but the most constant in the lower leg (**A9**) are near the posterior border of the tibia, one just below and one just above the medial malleolus (**A5**). The posterior arch vein (**A12**) unites these and perhaps other perforators and drains usually into the great saphenous vein below the knee.

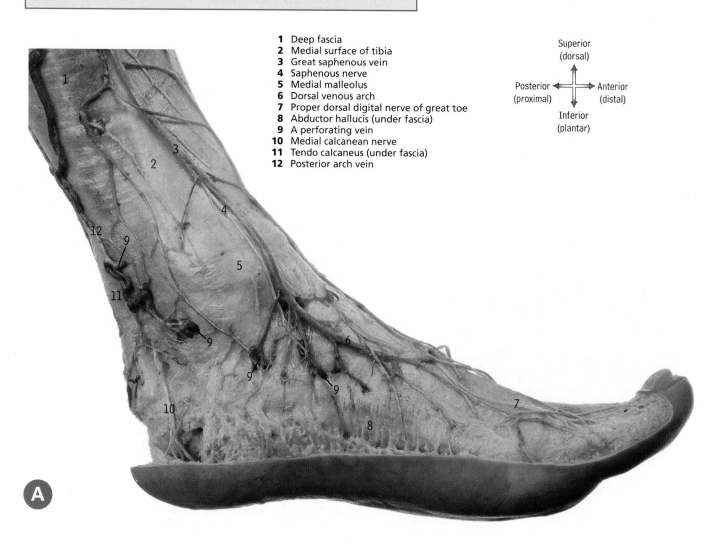

1 Deep fascia
2 Medial surface of tibia
3 Great saphenous vein
4 Saphenous nerve
5 Medial malleolus
6 Dorsal venous arch
7 Proper dorsal digital nerve of great toe
8 Abductor hallucis (under fascia)
9 A perforating vein
10 Medial calcanean nerve
11 Tendo calcaneus (under fascia)
12 Posterior arch vein

Superior
(dorsal)

Posterior ⟷ Anterior
(proximal)   (distal)

Inferior
(plantar)

A superficial vessels and nerves of the left lower leg and foot, from the medial side

The medial and lateral branches of the superficial fibular (*peroneal*) nerve (1 and 2) run on to the dorsum of the foot. Behind the lateral malleolus (7) are the small saphenous vein (5) and sural nerve (4). The tendon of fibularis (*peroneus*) longus (3) shines through the deep fascia above the malleolus.

- The superficial veins of the dorsum include dorsal digital and dorsal metatarsal veins, which join a dorsal venous arch (**B12**). The ends of the arch join medial and lateral marginal veins that run upward to become the great and small saphenous veins respectively. (In **A** there is no obvious medial marginal vein, but there is a lateral marginal vein in **B, 10**.)

- The deep veins run with the deep arteries. The larger arteries in the leg are usually accompanied by a pair of veins (venae commitantes).

- Lymph vessels, resembling narrow, thin-walled veins, accompany many arteries and veins, both superficial and deep. There are no lymph nodes in the foot; most of the lymphatic drainage of the lower limb is to inguinal nodes, but some lymphatic vessels drain into six or seven nodes that lie in the fat of the popliteal fossa. (Occasionally there is a single node beside the upper end of the anterior tibial artery in front of the interosseous membrane.)

---

 1 Medial branch of superficial fibular (*peroneal*) nerve
 2 Lateral branch of superficial fibular (*peroneal*) nerve
 3 Deep fascia over fibularis (*peroneus*) longus tendon
 4 Sural nerve
 5 Small saphenous vein
 6 Tendo calcaneus (under fascia)
 7 Lateral malleolus
 8 A perforating vein
 9 Extensor digitorum brevis (under fascia)
10 Lateral marginal vein
11 Abductor digiti minimi (under fascia)
12 Dorsal venous arch

Superior
(dorsal)

Lateral ⟵⟶ Medial
(left)

Inferior
(plantar)

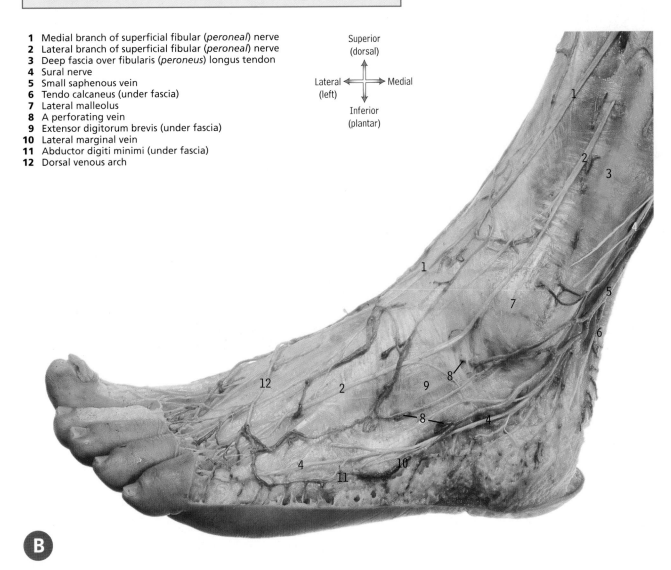

B

B superficial vessels and nerves of the left lower leg and foot, from the lateral side

Deep fascia of the foot

Deep fascia of the right lower leg and foot, from the front and the right

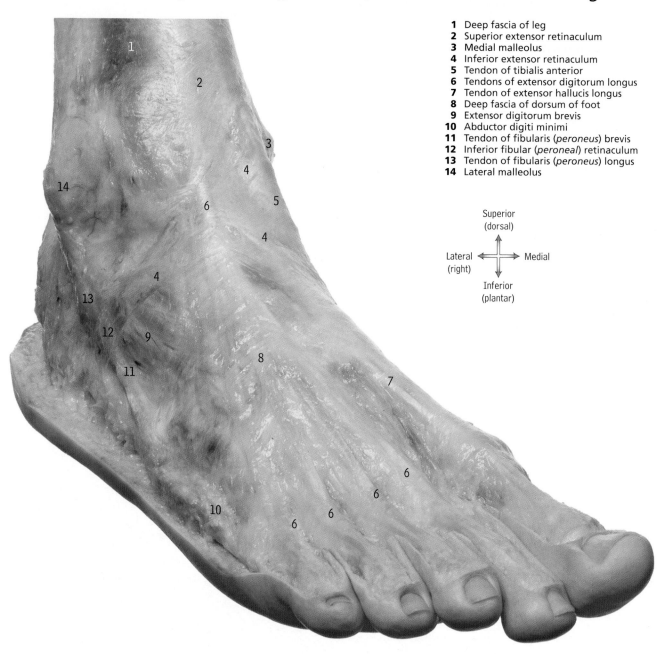

1 Deep fascia of leg
2 Superior extensor retinaculum
3 Medial malleolus
4 Inferior extensor retinaculum
5 Tendon of tibialis anterior
6 Tendons of extensor digitorum longus
7 Tendon of extensor hallucis longus
8 Deep fascia of dorsum of foot
9 Extensor digitorum brevis
10 Abductor digiti minimi
11 Tendon of fibularis (*peroneus*) brevis
12 Inferior fibular (*peroneal*) retinaculum
13 Tendon of fibularis (*peroneus*) longus
14 Lateral malleolus

Superior
(dorsal)

Lateral ←→ Medial
(right)

Inferior
(plantar)

All superficial tissues, including vessels and nerves, have been removed to display the deep fascia. It is thickened in places to form the retinacula (2, 4—see notes), which keep tendons in their proper places; compare with the dissections on pp. 74–77 where the fascia has been removed to leave only the retinacula. Here, with all the deep fascia intact, tendons and muscles can be seen shining through it.

- The retinacula of the ankle and foot are localized thickenings of deep fascia, which keep tendons in place.
- There are two extensor retinacula (superior and inferior), a flexor retinaculum and two fibular (*peroneal*) retinacula (superior and inferior).
- The superior extensor retinaculum (**2**) is a band about 4 cm broad, and is attached to the lower ends of the anterior borders of the tibia and fibula (see pp. 74, **A7** and 76, **A12**).
- The inferior extensor retinaculum (**4**) is shaped like a letter Y lying on its side (see pp. 74, **A9**; 76, **A15**; and 77, **B13**).

The common stem of the Y is on the lateral side and is attached to the upper surface of the calcaneus in front of the sulcus calcanei. The tendons of extensor digitorum longus and fibularis (*peroneus*) tertius (with a common synovial sheath) pass beneath it.

The upper band of the Y continues upward and medially from the common stem over the deep fibular (*peroneal*) nerve and anterior tibial vessels, then forms a loop to enclose the extensor hallucis longus tendon (within a synovial sheath), finally becoming attached to the medial malleolus after passing either superficial or deep to the tendon of tibialis anterior (within a synovial sheath).

The lower band of the Y continues downward and medially from the common stem, passing over the terminal branches of the deep fibular (*peroneal*) nerve, the dorsalis pedis vessels and the tendons of extensor hallucis longus (within a synovial sheath) and tibialis anterior, to blend with the plantar aponeurosis overlying abductor hallucis.

- For the flexor retinaculum, see p. 76.
- For the fibular (*peroneal*) retinacula, see p. 77.

Dorsum and back of the foot

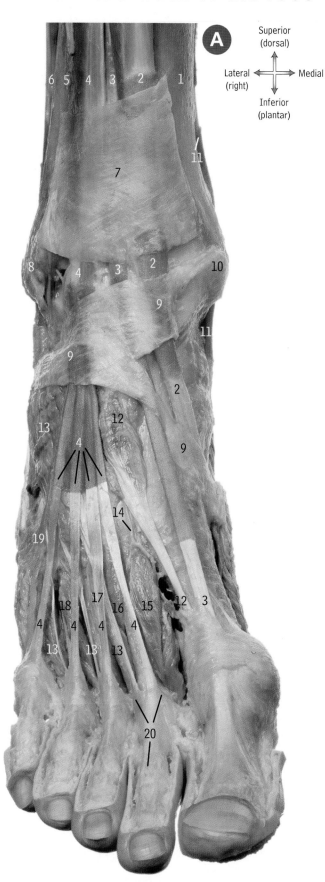

Superior
(dorsal)

Lateral ←→ Medial
(right)

Inferior
(plantar)

A superficial dissection of the right lower leg
and dorsum of the foot, from the front

Most of the deep fascia has been removed, leaving only
the retinacula (7 and 9). The most prominent structures
are the long tendons of the extensor muscles (2, 3 and
4) running down from the leg; the synovial sheaths
surrounding the tendons in this specimen (which is also
shown on pp. 76 and 77) have been emphasized by blue
tissue. Extensor digitorum brevis (13, with extensor
hallucis brevis, 12 — see notes) is the only muscle to
arise on the dorsum of the foot.

- Extensor digitorum longus (**4**) has four tendons that pass to the
  second, third, fourth and fifth toes.
- Extensor digitorum brevis (**13**) has four tendons that pass to the
  great, second, third and fourth toes. The part of the muscle that
  serves the great toe is known as extensor hallucis brevis (**12**).
- The dorsal digital expansions (extensor expansions, **20**) are
  derived from the tendons of extensor digitorum longus (**4**) as
  they pass over the metatarsophalangeal joints onto the dorsum
  of the proximal phalanges. They are each triangular in shape
  with the apex directed distally.

  On the second, third and fourth toes the basal angles of the
  expansions receive tendons from two interossei and one
  lumbrical muscle, and the central part of the base receives a
  tendon of extensor digitorum brevis (**13**). On the fifth toe one
  interosseus and one lumbrical tendon are attached.

  The central part of the apex is inserted into the base of the
  middle phalanx, while two collateral parts run farther forward
  to be inserted into the base of the distal phalanx (see p. 46,
  A16 and **17**).
- The order of the structures that pass beneath the superior
  extensor retinaculum and in front of the ankle joint from the
  medial to the lateral side is:

  Tibialis anterior tendon (with a synovial sheath) (**2**)
  Extensor hallucis longus tendon (with no synovial sheath) (**3**)
  Anterior tibial artery and venae comitantes ⎱ hidden between
  Deep fibular (*peroneal*) nerve   ⎰ **3** and **4**
  Extensor digitorum longus tendon (with no synovial sheath) (**4**)
  Fibularis (*peroneus*) tertius tendon (with no synovial sheath)
  (hidden by **4**)

1	Medial surface of tibia	
2	Tibialis anterior	
3	Extensor hallucis longus	
4	Extensor digitorum longus	
5	Subcutaneous surface of fibula	
6	Fibularis (*peroneus*) brevis	
7	Superior extensor retinaculum	
8	Lateral malleolus	
9	Inferior extensor retinaculum	
10	Medial malleolus	
11	Tibialis posterior	
12	Extensor hallucis brevis	
13	Extensor digitorum brevis	
14	Dorsalis pedis artery	
15	First dorsal interosseus	
16	Second dorsal interosseus	
17	Third dorsal interosseus	
18	Fourth dorsal interosseus	
19	Fibularis (*peroneus*) tertius	
20	Dorsal digital expansion	

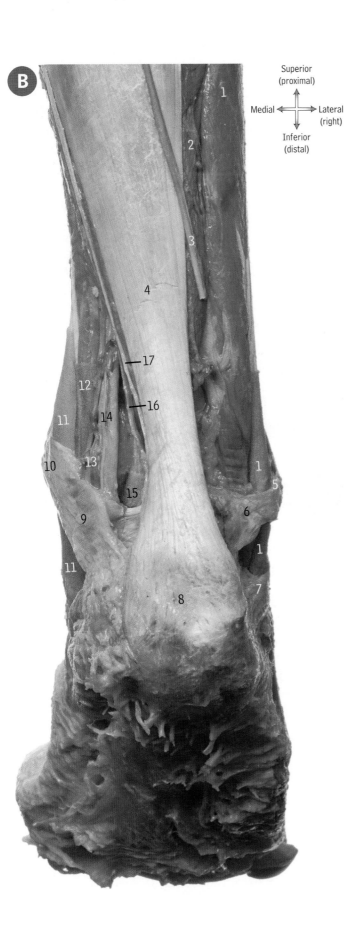

Superior
(proximal)

Medial ←——→ Lateral
(right)

Inferior
(distal)

B superficial dissection of the back of the right lower leg and foot

C palpation of the dorsalis pedis pulse. The dorsalis pedis pulse can be felt on a line from midway between the malleoli (5 and 10) toward the first toe cleft.

D palpation of the posterior tibial pulse. The posterior tibial pulse can be felt behind the medial malleolus (10) and 2.5 cm in front of the Achilles' tendon (4).

The deep fascia has been removed, leaving only the flexor and fibular (*peroneal*) retinacula (9, 6 and 7). The Achilles' tendon (4) passes down to the back of the calcaneus (8). Flexor tendons (11, 12 and 15) lie behind the medial malleolus (10) and fibular (*peroneal*) tendons (1) behind the lateral malleolus (5).

1 Fibularis (*peroneus*) longus overlapping fibularis (*peroneus*) brevis
2 Soleus
3 Sural nerve
4 Tendo calcaneus (Achilles' tendon)
5 Lateral malleolus
6 Superior fibular (*peroneal*) retinaculum
7 Inferior fibular (*peroneal*) retinaculum
8 Posterior surface of calcaneus
9 Flexor retinaculum
10 Medial malleolus
11 Tibialis posterior
12 Flexor digitorum longus
13 Posterior tibial artery and venae comitantes
14 Tibial nerve
15 Flexor hallucis longus
16 Medial calcanean nerve
17 Plantaris tendon

- For the order of the structures behind the medial malleolus, see the notes on the flexor retinaculum on p. 76.

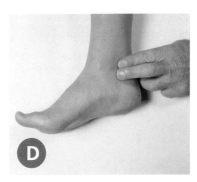

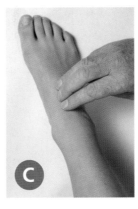

Dorsum and sides of the foot

The synovial sheaths of tendons have been emphasised by blue tissue. The deep fascia has been removed, leaving the flexor retinaculum (12), with part of the inferior extensor retinaculum (15) also visible in this view. The posterior tibial vessels (4) and the tibial nerve (5) lie between the tendons of flexor digitorum longus (3) in front and flexor hallucis longus (6) behind. The prominent muscle on the medial side of the sole is abductor hallucis (14).

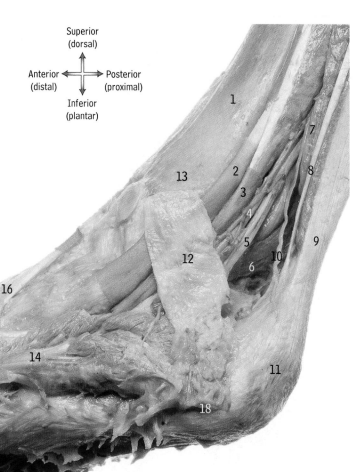

Superior
(dorsal)

Anterior ←→ Posterior
(distal)   (proximal)

Inferior
(plantar)

A superficial dissection of the right lower leg and foot, from the medial side.

1 Medial surface of tibia
2 Tibialis posterior
3 Flexor digitorum longus
4 Posterior tibial artery and venae comitantes
5 Tibial nerve
6 Flexor hallucis longus
7 Soleus
8 Plantaris tendon
9 Tendo calcaneus
10 Medial calcanean nerve
11 Posterior surface of calcaneus
12 Flexor retinaculum
13 Medial malleolus
14 Abductor hallucis
15 Inferior extensor retinaculum
16 Tibialis anterior
17 Extensor hallucis longus
18 Medial process of tuberosity of calcaneus

- The flexor retinaculum (12) passes from the medial malleolus to the medial process of the tuberosity of the calcaneus (18).

Deep to the retinaculum are four connective tissue compartments—three for tendons and one for neurovascular structures. The order of the structures behind the medial malleolus from before backwards is:

Tibialis posterior tendon (2, within a synovial sheath)
Flexor digitorum longus tendon (3, within a synovial sheath)
Posterior tibial artery and venae comitantes (4)
Tibial nerve (5)
Flexor hallucis longus tendon (6, within a synovial sheath).

The synovial sheaths of tendons have been emphasized by blue tissue. The two extensor retinacula (12 and 13) and the two fibular (*peroneal*) retinacula (14 and 15) have been preserved. The tendon of fibularis (*peroneus*) brevis (4) runs down to the fifth metatarsal, while that of fibularis (*peroneus*) longus (5) disappears to pass into the sole. Extensor digitorum brevis (16) forms a fleshy mass on the lateral side of the dorsum, and is crossed by the tendons of extensor digitorum longus (3) and fibularis (*peroneus*) tertius (17).

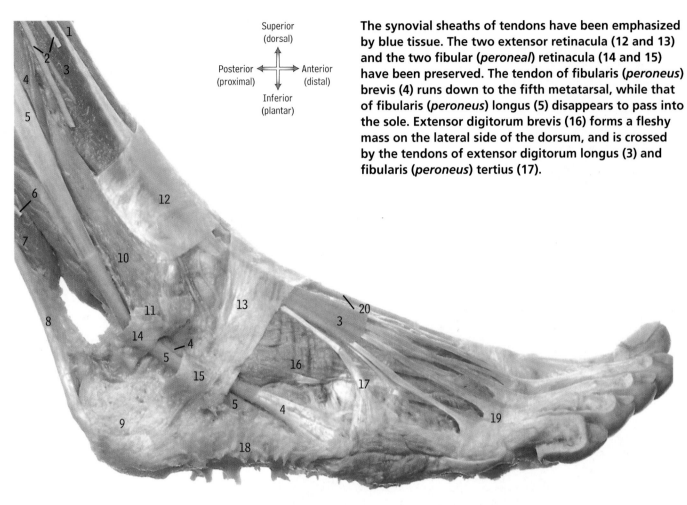

B superficial dissection of the right lower leg and foot, from the lateral side.

1 Tibialis anterior
2 Medial and lateral branches of superficial fibular (*peroneal*) nerve
3 Extensor digitorum longus
4 Fibularis (*peroneus*) brevis
5 Fibularis (*peroneus*) longus
6 Sural nerve
7 Soleus
8 Tendo calcaneus
9 Lateral surface of calcaneus
10 Subcutaneous area of fibula
11 Lateral malleolus
12 Superior extensor retinaculum
13 Inferior extensor retinaculum
14 Superior fibular (*peroneal*) retinaculum
15 Inferior fibular (*peroneal*) retinaculum
16 Extensor digitorum brevis
17 Fibularis (*peroneus*) tertius
18 Abductor digiti minimi
19 A dorsal digital expansion
20 Extensor hallucis longus

- The superior fibular (*peroneal*) retinaculum (**14**) passes from the lateral malleolus (**11**) to the lateral surface of the calcaneus (**9**).

  Deep to the retinaculum are the tendons of fibularis (*peroneus*) brevis (**4**) and fibularis (*peroneus*) longus (**5**) (both within a single synovial sheath). The brevis tendon is in front of the longus tendon.

- The inferior fibular (*peroneal*) retinaculum (**15**) continues backwards and downwards from the common stem of the inferior extensor retinaculum (**13**) to the lateral surface of the calcaneus (**9**), with an intermediate attachment to the fibular (*peroneal*) trochlea (see p. 60, **D9**).

  Deep to the retinaculum above and in front of the trochlea is the fibularis (*peroneus*) brevis tendon (**4**, within its own synovial sheath), while below and behind the trochlea is the fibularis (*peroneus*) longus tendon (**5**, within its own synovial sheath).

Dorsum and sides of the foot

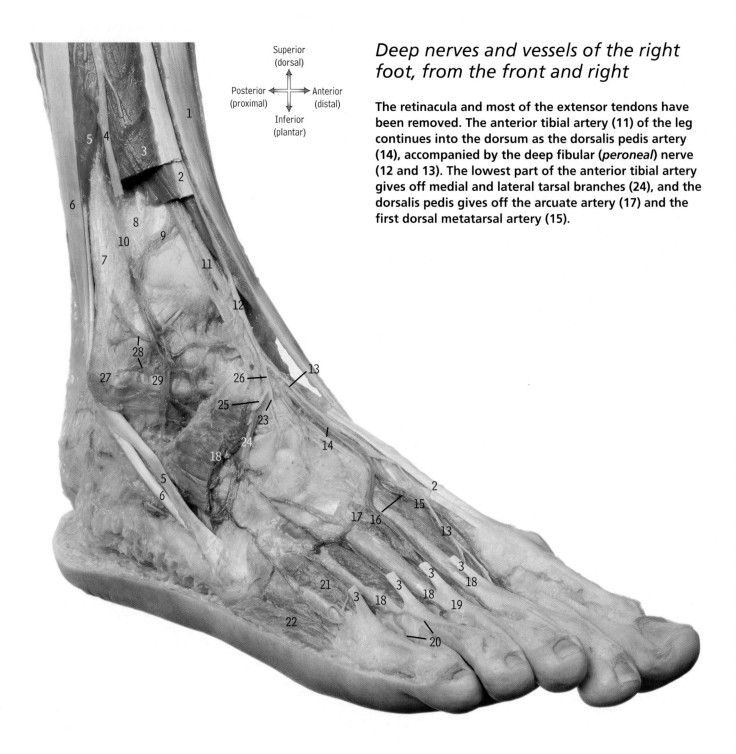

Superior
(dorsal)

Posterior ◄━━━► Anterior
(proximal)   (distal)

Inferior
(plantar)

Deep nerves and vessels of the right foot, from the front and right

The retinacula and most of the extensor tendons have been removed. The anterior tibial artery (11) of the leg continues into the dorsum as the dorsalis pedis artery (14), accompanied by the deep fibular (*peroneal*) nerve (12 and 13). The lowest part of the anterior tibial artery gives off medial and lateral tarsal branches (24), and the dorsalis pedis gives off the arcuate artery (17) and the first dorsal metatarsal artery (15).

1 Tibialis anterior
2 Extensor hallucis longus
3 Extensor digitorum longus
4 Lateral branch of superficial fibular (*peroneal*) nerve
5 Fibularis (*peroneus*) brevis
6 Fibularis (*peroneus*) longus
7 Subcutaneous surface of fibula
8 Interosseous membrane
9 Lateral malleolar artery and venae comitantes
10 Perforating branch of fibular (*peroneal*) artery
11 Anterior tibial vessels
12 Deep fibular (*peroneal*) nerve
13 Medial terminal branch of **12**
14 Dorsalis pedis artery
15 First dorsal metatarsal artery

16 Deep plantar artery
17 Arcuate artery
18 Extensor digitorum brevis (hallucis brevis to great toe)
19 Dorsal digital expansion
20 Dorsal digital artery
21 Fourth dorsal interosseus
22 Abductor digiti minimi
23 Interosseous branch of **26**
24 Lateral tarsal vessels
25 Nerve to extensor digitorum brevis
26 Lateral terminal branch of **12**
27 Lateral malleolus
28 Lateral malleolar arterial rete
29 Anterior talofibular ligament

- As the anterior tibial artery (**11**) crosses the lower margin of the tibia at the ankle joint it becomes the dorsalis pedis artery (**14**).

- After giving off medial and lateral tarsal branches (**24**) the dorsalis pedis artery (**14**) ends by dividing into the first dorsal metatarsal and the arcuate arteries (**15** and **17**).

- The first dorsal metatarsal artery (**15**) gives off a deep plantar (perforating) branch (**16**) that passes into the sole between the two heads of the first dorsal interosseus muscle to complete the plantar arch with the deep part of the lateral plantar artery (see p. 87, **B18**).

- The arcuate artery (**17**) gives off the other three dorsal metatarsal arteries,

and all the metatarsal arteries give dorsal digital branches.

- Sometimes the perforating branch of the fibular (*peroneal*) artery (**10**), which anastomoses with the lateral tarsal and arcuate arteries (**24** and **17**), is large and replaces the dorsalis pedis artery, which is absent in about 12% of feet.

- Theoretically each side of each toe has a dorsal digital artery and a plantar digital artery but the individual vessels soon become merged into an anastomotic network.

- For a summary of the branches of the dorsalis pedis artery see p. 123.

Deep dissection of the dorsum
Joints beneath the talus of the left foot

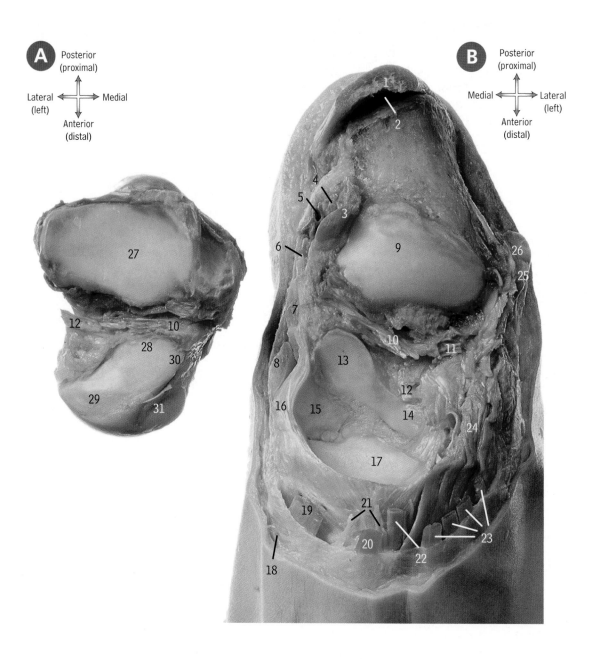

A

Posterior
(proximal)

Lateral
(left) ←→ Medial

Anterior
(distal)

B

Posterior
(proximal)

Medial ←→ Lateral
(left)

Anterior
(distal)

The talus has been removed from the left foot and turned upside down to lie adjacent, so exposing the reciprocal joint surfaces. At the back the concave posterior articular surface of the talus (27) forms the talocalcanean joint with the convex posterior articular surface of the calcaneus (9). At the front are the various parts of the talocalcaneonavicular joint (see notes). The convex middle and anterior surfaces of the talus (28 and 29) articulate with the concave middle and anterior surfaces of the calcaneus (13 and 14), with part of the anterior surface of the talus (30) articulating with cartilage in the upper surface of the spring ligament (15). The convex head of the talus (31) articulates with the concave posterior surface of the navicular bone (17).

1　Tendo calcaneus
2　Bursa
3　Flexor hallucis longus
4　Lateral plantar nerve
5　Posterior tibial vessels
6　Medial plantar nerve
7　Flexor digitorum longus
8　Tibialis posterior
9　Posterior articular surface of calcaneus
10　Interosseous talocalcanean ligament
11　Inferior extensor retinaculum
12　Cervical ligament
13　Middle ⎫
14　Anterior ⎬ articular surface of calcaneus
15　Cartilage in plantar calcaneonavicular (spring) ligament
16　Medial (deltoid) ligament of ankle joint
17　Posterior articular surface of navicular
18　Great saphenous vein
19　Tibialis anterior
20　Extensor hallucis longus
21　Deep fibular (*peroneal*) nerve
22　Dorsalis pedis artery
23　Extensor digitorum longus
24　Extensor digitorum brevis
25　Fibularis (*peroneus*) brevis
26　Fibularis (*peroneus*) longus
27　Posterior ⎫
28　Middle ⎬ calcanean articular surface of talus
29　Anterior ⎭
30　Surface for plantar calcaneonavicular (spring) ligament
31　Surface for navicular

- Apart from the joints of the toes, the most important joints of the rest of the foot are those related to the talus.

- Above the talus is the ankle joint (properly known as the talocrural joint), between the trochlear surface of the talus and the lower ends of the tibia and fibula.

- Below the talus there are two separate joints. Towards the back is the talocalcanean joint (alternatively known as the subtalar joint — but see below), between the posterior articular surfaces of the lower part of the talus (27) and upper part of the calcaneus (9). In front is the talocalcaneonavicular joint, which is a two-part joint between the front of the head of the talus (31) and the navicular (17) (the talonavicular part of this joint), and the articulations of the undersurface of the talus (28–30) with the anterior and middle facets on the upper surface of the calcaneus (14 and 13) and the upper surface of the plantar calcaneonavicular (spring) ligament (15) (the talocalcanean part of this joint).

- Unfortunately there is some confusion of terminology, for clinicians frequently use 'subtalar joint' as a collective name for *both* joints beneath the talus, not just the posterior one.

Sole of the foot
Plantar aponeurosis of the left foot

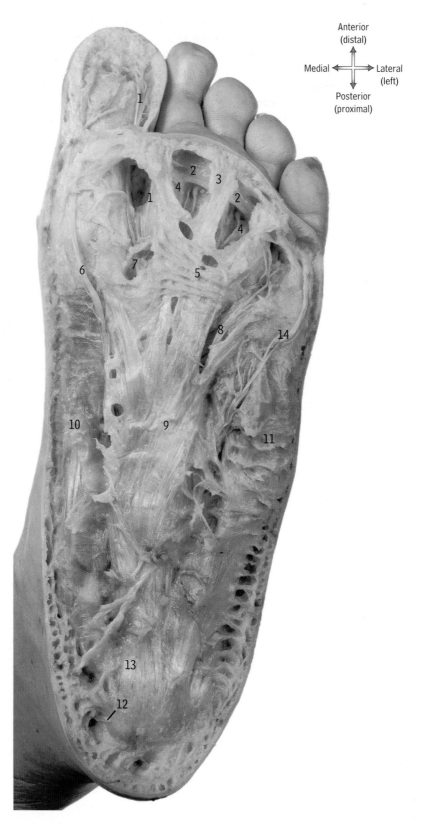

Skin and subcutaneous tissue have been removed to show the thick central part of the plantar aponeurosis (9) and the thinner medial and lateral parts (10 and 11). The numerous strands and septa of fibrous tissue that attach the aponeurosis to the overlying tissues have not been removed to make a tidy dissection; they are an important part of the anatomy of the sole, binding adjacent tissues together.

- **Nerve supplies** in the sole include the following:

  Cutaneous: the medial plantar nerve supplies the medial part of the sole and the medial three and a half toes; the lateral plantar nerve supplies the lateral part of the sole and lateral one and a half toes.

  Muscular: the medial plantar nerve supplies abductor hallucis, flexor hallucis brevis, flexor digitorum brevis and the first lumbrical; the lateral plantar nerve supplies all the other small muscles of the sole.

  For details of nerve branches see pp. 121 and 122.

- The skin under the heel and on the lateral part of the sole is part of the first sacral dermatome, with the fifth lumbar dermatome including the rest of the sole (**Fig. 9**, p. 121).

- The superficial surface of the plantar aponeurosis is not smooth as in most textbook drawings, but roughened by the attachment of numerous fibrous septa forming loculations that hold the fatty subcutaneous tissues and skin in place when weight-bearing. They are well shown toward the back and sides of the dissection illustrated here.

---

1 Plantar digital nerve
2 Superficial transverse metatarsal ligament
3 Superficial layer of digital band of aponeurosis
4 Deep layer of digital band of aponeurosis
5 Transverse fibres of aponeurosis
6 Proper plantar digital nerve of great toe
7 Common plantar digital branch of medial plantar nerve
8 Common plantar digital branch of lateral plantar nerve
9 Central part of aponeurosis overlying flexor digitorum brevis
10 Medial part of aponeurosis overlying abductor hallucis
11 Lateral part of aponeurosis overlying abductor digiti minimi
12 Medial calcanean nerve
13 Medial process of tuberosity of calcaneus
14 Proper plantar digital nerve of fifth toe

Sole of the foot

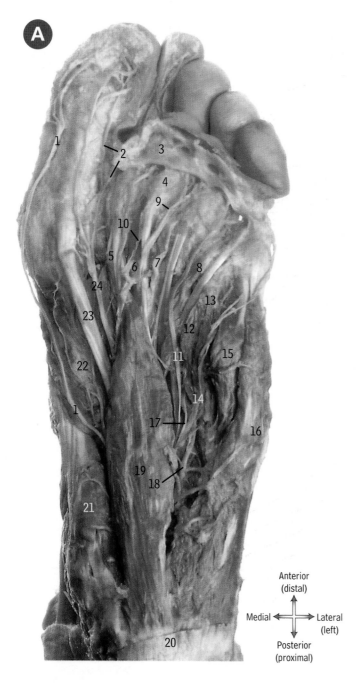

A first layer of muscles of the left sole

The plantar aponeurosis has been removed. The central muscle is flexor digitorum brevis (19), with abductor hallucis (21) on the medial side and abductor digiti minimi (16) on the lateral side. The most prominent tendon is that of flexor hallucis longus (23). Digital branches of the medial and lateral plantar nerves (1, 2, 10, 11 and 14) run forward towards the toes, and the deep branch of the lateral plantar nerve (17), which supplies many of the deeper muscles, curves deeply into the sole. See also Fig. 4, p. 120.

- The muscles of the sole are usually classified in **four layers**, as seen in progressively deep dissection:

  First layer: abductor hallucis (**A21**), flexor digitorum brevis (**A19**) and abductor digiti minimi (**A16**).

  Second layer: Quadratus plantae (**B19**) and the four lumbrical muscles (**B7–10**), with the tendons of flexor digitorum longus (**B4**) and flexor hallucis longus (**B1**).

  Third layer: flexor hallucis brevis (p. 86, **A8**), adductor hallucis (p. 86, **A6** and **7**) and flexor digiti minimi brevis (p. 86, **A14**).

  Fourth layer: three plantar and four dorsal interosseus muscles (p. 87, **B5–11**), with the tendons of tibialis posterior (p. 87, **B27**) and fibularis (*peroneus*) longus (p. 87, **B24**).

  The successive layers do not completely obscure one another; for example, the third plantar and fourth dorsal interossei (**A13** and **12**) are seen as soon as the plantar aponeurosis has been removed. (The layers refer to layers of *muscles*; the plantar aponeurosis is not itself the first layer but overlies it.)

- It may be functionally more useful to classify the muscles into **medial**, **lateral** *and* **intermediate** *groups*:

  Medial group, for the great toe: abductor hallucis, flexor hallucis brevis, adductor hallucis and the tendon of flexor hallucis longus.

  Lateral group, for the fifth toe: abductor digiti minimi and flexor digiti minimi brevis.

  Intermediate group, for the second to fifth toes: flexor digitorum brevis, quadratus plantae, the tendons of flexor digitorum longus and the lumbricals, and the interossei.

Anterior
(distal)

Medial ◄———► Lateral
(left)

Posterior
(proximal)

1 Proper plantar digital nerve of great toe	**13** Third plantar interosseus
2 Proper plantar digital nerves of first cleft	**14** Proper plantar digital nerve of fifth toe
3 Superficial transverse metatarsal ligament	**15** Flexor digiti minimi brevis
4 Fibrous flexor sheath	**16** Abductor digiti minimi
5 First lumbrical	**17** Deep branch of lateral plantar nerve
6 Second lumbrical	**18** Lateral plantar artery
7 Third lumbrical	**19** Flexor digitorum brevis
8 Fourth lumbrical	**20** Plantar aponeurosis
9 Third plantar metatarsal artery	**21** Abductor hallucis
10 A superficial digital branch of medial plantar artery	**22** Flexor hallucis brevis
11 Fourth common plantar digital nerve	**23** Flexor hallucis longus
12 Fourth dorsal interosseus	**24** First common plantar digital nerve

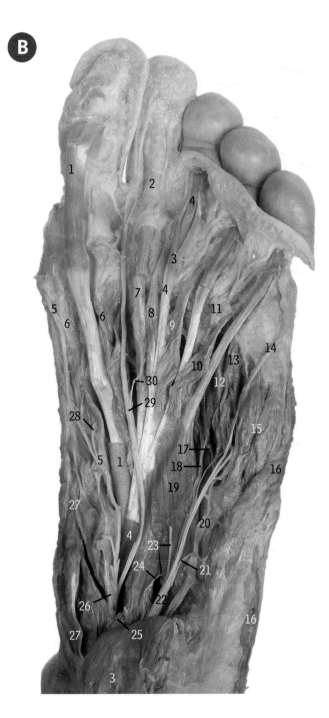

B second layer of muscles of the left sole

Flexor digitorum brevis has been removed (but the abductors of the great and little toes, 27 and 16, remain) to display quadratus plantae (19) joining flexor digitorum longus (4) as it divides into its four tendons, from which the lumbrical muscles arise (7–10). The deep branch of the lateral plantar nerve (18) curls round the lateral side of quadratus plantae (19) to reach the deeper part of the sole, and numerous other muscular and digital (cutaneous) branches of the medial and lateral plantar nerves (26 and 22) are visible. Synovial sheaths of flexor tendons have been emphasized by blue tissue. See also Fig. 5, p. 120.

- Although flexor hallucis longus (**B1**) passes to the great toe on the *medial* side of the foot, it arises from the *fibula* on the lateral side of the leg. The tendon crosses over in the sole, deep to flexor digitorum longus (**B4**, toward the back of the sole).

- The lateral and medial plantar nerves and vessels (**B20, 22** and **26**) pass between the first and second layers of muscles. The deep branch of the lateral plantar nerve (**A17, B18**) and the deep branch of the artery, which becomes the lateral plantar arch (**B17**), curl deeply round the lateral border of quadratus plantae (**B19**).

1 Flexor hallucis longus
2 Fibrous flexor sheath
3 Flexor digitorum brevis
4 Flexor digitorum longus
5 Proper plantar digital nerve of great toe
6 Flexor hallucis brevis
7 First lumbrical
8 Second lumbrical
9 Third lumbrical
10 Fourth lumbrical
11 Fourth plantar metatarsal artery
12 Fourth dorsal interosseus
13 Third plantar interosseus
14 Proper plantar digital nerve of fifth toe
15 Flexor digiti minimi brevis
16 Abductor digiti minimi
17 Plantar arch
18 Deep branch of lateral plantar nerve
19 Quadratus plantae
20 Lateral plantar artery
21 Nerve to abductor digiti minimi
22 Lateral plantar nerve
23 Fourth common plantar digital nerve
24 Nerve to quadratus plantae
25 Nerve to flexor digitorum brevis
26 Medial plantar artery overlying nerve
27 Abductor hallucis
28 Nerve to flexor hallucis brevis
29 First common plantar digital nerve
30 Nerve to first lumbrical

Sole of the foot

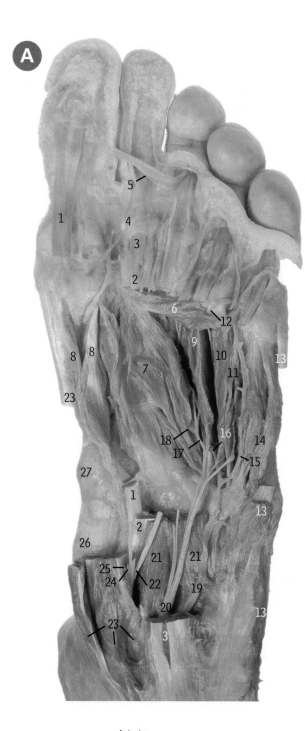

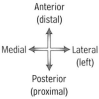

Anterior
(distal)

Medial ◄─────► Lateral
(left)

Posterior
(proximal)

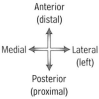

A third layer of muscles of the left sole

Most of the flexors and abductors have been removed, displaying the two heads of adductor hallucis (6 and 7), flexor hallucis brevis (8, which divides to pass to either side of the great toe), flexor digiti minimi brevis (14) and interossei (9–11). The deep branch of the lateral plantar nerve (17) is accompanied by the plantar arch (16) (from the lateral plantar artery, 19). See also Fig. 6, p. 121.

- For a summary of the medial and lateral plantar nerves see pp. 122 and 123.
- The third common plantar digital nerve (from the medial plantar nerve) frequently has a communicating branch with the (fourth) common plantar digital branch of the lateral plantar nerve, but it was not present in the specimens dissected here.
- Branches of the lateral plantar nerve (**A20, B21**) to various interosseus muscles (**A9–11, B5–11**) can be seen but have been left unlabeled.
- The plantar arch (**B18**) is the deep continuation of the lateral plantar artery (**B20**), which is the larger terminal branch of the posterior tibial artery. The arch is completed by anastomosis with the deep plantar (perforating) branch of the first dorsal metatarsal artery (see p. 78, **15**).
  The arch gives off four plantar metatarsal arteries (as in **B15** and **16**), which divide to give plantar digital branches to the sides of adjacent toes. There are separate branches for the medial side of the great toe and lateral side of the fifth toe.
- The medial plantar artery (**A24, B23**), smaller than the lateral and subject to considerable variation, does not take part directly in the formation of the arch. It usually anastomoses with the plantar digital branch to the medial side of the great toe, and gives off superficial digital branches that anastomose with the first three plantar metatarsal arteries.

1 Flexor hallucis longus
2 Flexor digitorum longus
3 Flexor digitorum brevis
4 Fibrous flexor sheath
5 Long vinculum
6 Transverse head ⎫ of adductor hallucis
7 Oblique head   ⎭
8 Flexor hallucis brevis
9 Second plantar interosseus
10 Fourth dorsal interosseus
11 Third plantar interosseus
12 Fourth plantar metatarsal artery
13 Abductor digiti minimi
14 Flexor digiti minimi brevis
15 Nerve to flexor digiti minimi brevis
16 Plantar arch
17 Deep branch of lateral plantar nerve
18 Nerve to adductor hallucis
19 Lateral plantar artery
20 Lateral plantar nerve
21 Quadratus plantae
22 Medial plantar nerve
23 Abductor hallucis
24 Medial plantar artery
25 Nerve to abductor hallucis
26 Tuberosity of navicular
27 Tibialis anterior

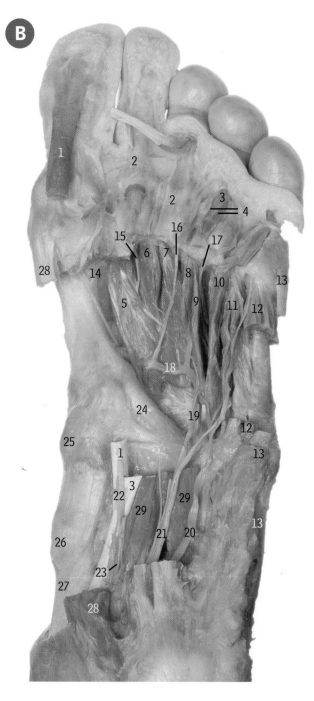

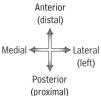

Anterior
(distal)

Medial ←——+——→ Lateral
(left)

Posterior
(proximal)

B fourth layer of muscles of the left sole

Most of the smaller muscles have been removed, leaving only the three plantar interossei (7, 9 and 11) and the four dorsal interossei (5, 6, 8 and 10). The tendon of tibialis posterior (27) passes mainly to the tuberosity of the navicular (26), and the tendon of fibularis (*peroneus*) longus (24) crosses the sole obliquely from the lateral to the medial side. The end of the synovial sheath of flexor hallucis longus (1) has been emphasized by blue tissue. See also Fig. 7, p. 121.

- Viewed from the sole, both plantar *and* dorsal interossei (**B5–11**) are visible; they lie side by side, not (as might be expected from their names) with the plantar group completely overlying and obscuring the dorsal. (But, on the dorsum only dorsal interossei are seen between the metatarsals — as on p. 74, **A15–18**.)
  The *plantar* interossei *ad*duct toes and the *dorsal* interossei *ab*duct them at the metatarsophalangeal joints, the reference line or axis for these movements being the line of the second toe. The mnemonics PAD and DAB are the usual aids to recalling which group does what.
  The great toe and the fifth toe each have their own abductor muscle; the great toe also has its own adductor to draw it nearer the second toe. It follows that there must be a plantar interosseus for each of the third, fourth and fifth toes so that they can be adducted toward the axial line.
  The second toe has no plantar interosseus but it has two dorsal interossei, one on each side so that it can be abducted to either side of its own neutral position. The third and fourth toes both have one of each interosseus.

- For other and probably more important actions of the interossei see p. 99.

- For a summary of the medial and lateral plantar arteries see p. 122.

1 Flexor hallucis longus
2 Fibrous flexor sheath
3 Flexor digitorum longus
4 Flexor digitorum brevis
5 First dorsal ⎫
6 Second dorsal ⎪
7 First plantar ⎪
8 Third dorsal ⎬ interosseus
9 Second plantar ⎪
10 Fourth dorsal ⎪
11 Third plantar ⎭
12 Flexor digiti minimi brevis
13 Abductor digiti minimi
14 First plantar metatarsal artery
15 Second plantar metatarsal artery
16 Third plantar metatarsal artery
17 Fourth plantar metatarsal artery
18 Plantar arch
19 Deep branch of lateral plantar nerve
20 Lateral plantar artery
21 Lateral plantar nerve
22 Medial plantar nerve
23 Medial plantar artery
24 Fibularis (*peroneus*) longus
25 Tibialis anterior
26 Tuberosity of navicular
27 Tibialis posterior
28 Abductor hallucis
29 Quadratus plantae

Ligaments of the foot *ligaments of the right foot*

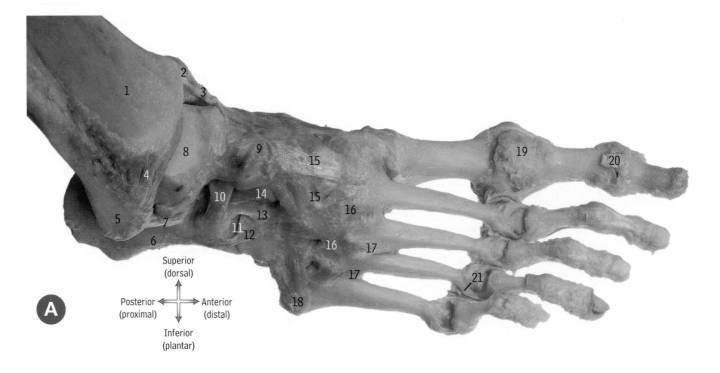

A

Superior
(dorsal)

Posterior ← → Anterior
(proximal) (distal)

Inferior
(plantar)

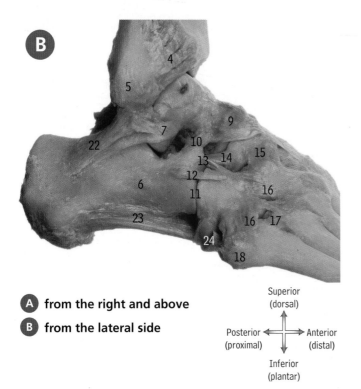

B

Ⓐ **from the right and above**

Ⓑ **from the lateral side**

Superior
(dorsal)

Posterior ← → Anterior
(proximal) (distal)

Inferior
(plantar)

1 Tibia
2 Medial malleolus
3 Medial (deltoid) ligament of ankle joint
4 Anterior tibiofibular ligament
5 Lateral malleolus
6 Calcaneus
7 Anterior talofibular ligament
8 Trochlear surface of talus (ankle joint capsule removed)
9 Head of talus (under capsule of talonavicular part of talocalcaneonavicular joint)
10 Cervical ligament
11 Calcaneocuboid joint
12 Dorsal calcaneocuboid ligament
13 Calcaneocuboid part ⎫ of bifurcate ligament
14 Calcaneonavicular part ⎭
15 Dorsal cuneonavicular ligaments
16 Dorsal tarsometatarsal ligaments
17 Dorsal metatarsal ligaments
18 Tuberosity of base of fifth metatarsal
19 Capsule of first metatarsophalangeal joint
20 Tendon of extensor hallucis longus
21 Collateral ligament
22 Calcaneofibular ligament
23 Long plantar ligament
24 Tendon of fibularis (*peroneus*) longus
25 Interosseous membrane
26 Posterior tibiofibular ligament
27 Tibial slip of 28
28 Posterior talofibular ligament
29 Groove for flexor hallucis longus tendon on talus and sustentaculum tali
30 Posterior tibiotalar part ⎫ of medial deltoid ligament
31 Tibiocalcanean part (deltoid) ⎭
32 Groove for tibialis posterior tendon
33 Groove for fibularis (*peroneus*) brevis tendon

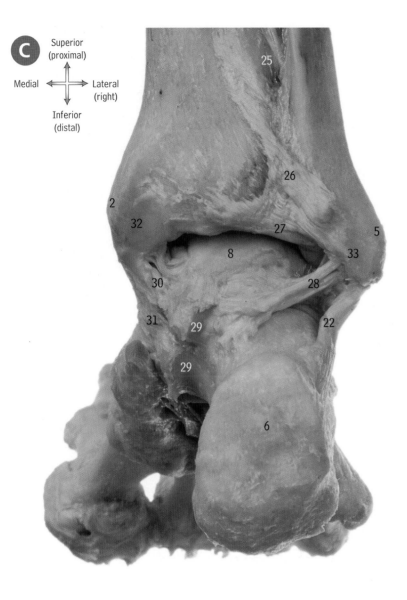

C Superior (proximal)

Medial ← → Lateral (right)

Inferior (distal)

C from behind

In A the foot is plantarflexed, showing part of the trochlear (superior articular) surface of the talus (8), with the front of the deltoid ligament (3) on the medial side and the anterior tibiofibular ligament (4) on the lateral side. The cervical ligament (10) passes upward and medially from the upper surface of the calcaneus to the undersurface of the talus, and in front of it are the two parts of the bifurcate ligament (13 and 14) with a small dorsal calcaneocuboid ligament (12) more laterally. Other dorsal ligaments (15, 16 and 17) connect adjacent bones.

In B the anterior talofibular ligament (7) and calcaneofibular ligament (22) are seen, with some of the smaller dorsal ligaments (12–17), and so is the posterior part of the long plantar ligament (23) in the sole.

In C the posterior talofibular ligament (28) runs transversely (so it is not seen in the lateral view in B); it has a tibial slip (27) which merges with the inferior transverse ligament, the name given to the lower part of the posterior tibiofibular ligament (26).

On the medial side of the ankle joint there is a single medial (deltoid) ligament (**A3**) (although it has several parts, as on p. 90, **A2–5**), but on the lateral side there is no single lateral ligament but three separate ligaments: the anterior and posterior talofibular ligaments (**A7** and **B7, C28**) and the calcaneofibular ligament (**B22** and **C22**).

Ligaments of the foot

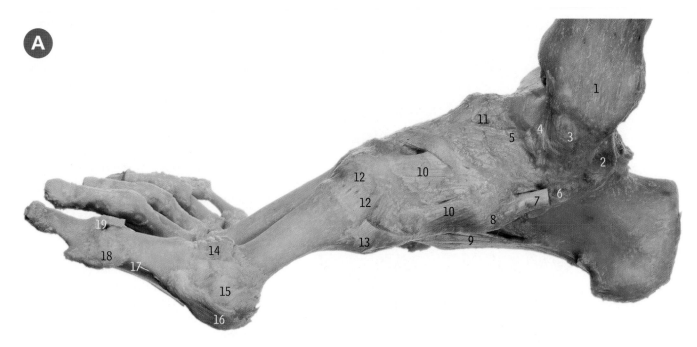

A ligaments of the right foot, from the medial side

On the medial side of the ankle the various parts of the medial (deltoid) ligament (2–5) merge with one another. The tendon of tibialis posterior (7) is mainly attached to the tuberosity of the navicular (8), while that of tibialis anterior (13) runs to the medial cuneiform and the base of the first metatarsal.

1	Medial malleolus
2	Posterior tibiotalar part ⎫
3	Tibiocalcanean part ⎬ of medial (deltoid) ligament
4	Anterior tibiotalar part ⎬
5	Tibionavicular part ⎭
6	Sustentaculum tali
7	Tibialis posterior
8	Tuberosity of navicular
9	Long plantar ligament
10	Dorsal cuneonavicular ligament

11	Talonavicular ligament
12	Dorsal ligaments of first tarsometatarsal joint
13	Tibialis anterior
14	Capsule ⎫ of first metatarsophalangeal joint
15	Collateral ligament ⎭
16	Sesamoid bone
17	Flexor hallucis longus
18	Collateral ligament of interphalangeal joint
19	Extensor hallucis longus

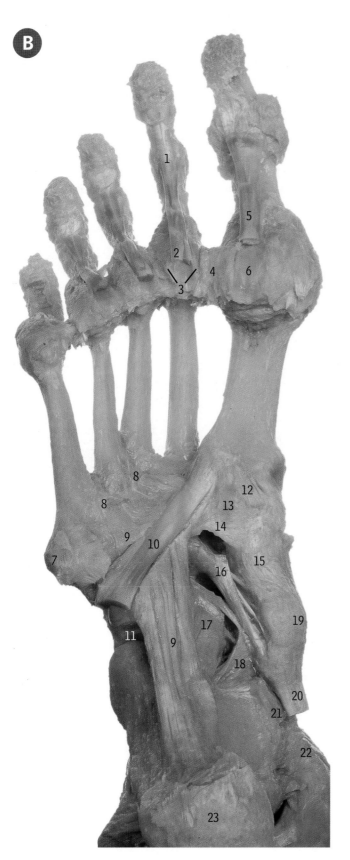

B Ligaments of the sole of the right foot

Part of the long plantar ligament (9) has been cut away to show the tendon of fibularis (*peroneus*) longus (10) lying in the groove on the cuboid. Medial to the posterior part of the long plantar ligament is the short plantar (plantar calcaneocuboid) ligament (17), and medial to that is the spring (plantar calcaneonavicular) ligament (18). At the anterior part of the foot the deep transverse metatarsal ligaments (4) keep the heads of the metatarsals and the bases of the toes from spreading apart.

1 Flexor digitorum longus
2 Flexor digitorum brevis
3 Fibrous flexor sheath
4 Deep transverse metatarsal ligament
5 Flexor hallucis longus
6 Plantar ligament of first tarsometatarsal joint
7 Tuberosity of base of fifth metatarsal
8 Plantar metatarsal ligaments
9 Long plantar ligament
10 Tendon of fibularis (*peroneus*) longus in groove on cuboid
11 Calcaneocuboid joint
12 Plantar tarsometatarsal ligament
13 Medial cuneiform
14 Cuneometatarsal ligament
15 Plantar cuneonavicular ligament
16 Fibrous slip from tibialis posterior overlying a cuneometatarsal ligament
17 Plantar calcaneocuboid (short plantar) ligament
18 Plantar calcaneonavicular (spring) ligament
19 Tuberosity of navicular
20 Tendon of tibialis posterior
21 Sustentaculum tali and groove for flexor hallucis longus
22 Medial (deltoid) ligament of ankle joint
23 Tuberosity of calcaneus

- The *medial* sides of the medial cuneiform and the base of the first metatarsal receive the attachment of the tibialis anterior tendon (**A13**); the *lateral* sides of the same two bones receive the attachment of the fibularis (*peroneus*) longus tendon (**B10**).

- The plantar calcaneocuboid ligament (**B17**), commonly called the short plantar ligament, is largely under cover of the long plantar ligament (**B9**), which with the groove on the cuboid bone forms an osseofibrous tunnel for the fibularis (*peroneus*) longus tendon (**B10**).

- The plantar calcaneonavicular ligament (**B18**), passing from the sustentaculum tali of the calcaneus to the navicular and commonly called the spring ligament although it is not elastic, is an important support for the head of the talus in the talocalcaneonavicular joint (p. 81, **15**).

Sections of the foot *sagittal sections of the right foot*

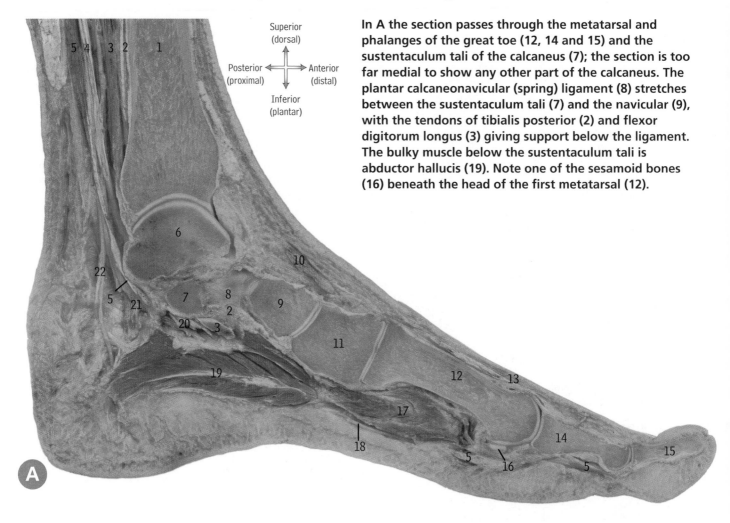

In A the section passes through the metatarsal and phalanges of the great toe (12, 14 and 15) and the sustentaculum tali of the calcaneus (7); the section is too far medial to show any other part of the calcaneus. The plantar calcaneonavicular (spring) ligament (8) stretches between the sustentaculum tali (7) and the navicular (9), with the tendons of tibialis posterior (2) and flexor digitorum longus (3) giving support below the ligament. The bulky muscle below the sustentaculum tali is abductor hallucis (19). Note one of the sesamoid bones (16) beneath the head of the first metatarsal (12).

A through the medial part of the talus, sustentaculum tali of the calcaneus and the great toe, from the lateral side

1 Tibia
2 Tibialis posterior
3 Flexor digitorum longus
4 Tibial nerve
5 Flexor hallucis longus
6 Talus
7 Sustentaculum tali
8 Plantar calcaneonavicular (spring) ligament
9 Navicular
10 Tibialis anterior

11 Medial cuneiform
12 First metatarsal
13 Extensor hallucis longus
14 Proximal phalanx
15 Distal phalanx
16 Sesamoid bone
17 Flexor hallucis brevis
18 Proper plantar digital nerve of great toe
19 Abductor hallucis
20 Medial plantar nerve and vessels

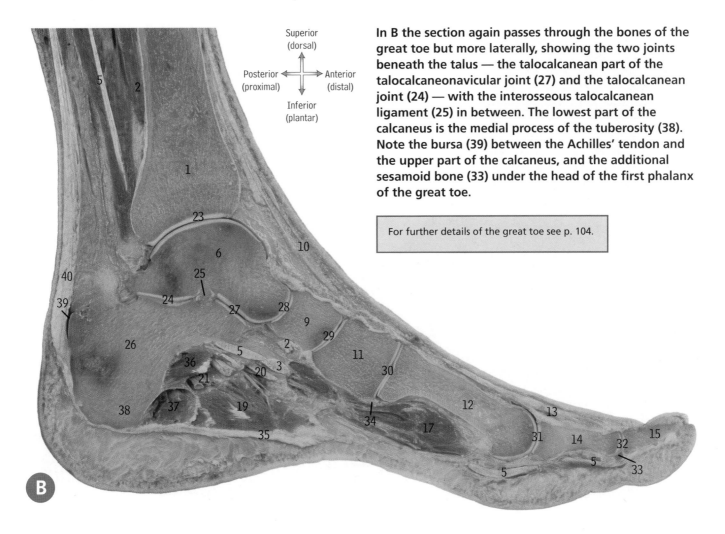

In B the section again passes through the bones of the great toe but more laterally, showing the two joints beneath the talus — the talocalcanean part of the talocalcaneonavicular joint (27) and the talocalcanean joint (24) — with the interosseous talocalcanean ligament (25) in between. The lowest part of the calcaneus is the medial process of the tuberosity (38). Note the bursa (39) between the Achilles' tendon and the upper part of the calcaneus, and the additional sesamoid bone (33) under the head of the first phalanx of the great toe.

For further details of the great toe see p. 104.

B through the center of the talus, medial part of the calcaneus and the great toe, from the lateral side (in a different foot from that in A)

21 Lateral plantar nerve and vessels	**31** Metatarsophalangeal joint
22 Medial calcanean nerve	**32** Interphalangeal joint
23 Ankle joint	**33** Additional sesamoid bone
24 Talocalcanean joint	**34** Fibularis (*peroneus*) longus
25 Interosseous talocalcanean ligament	**35** Plantar aponeurosis
26 Calcaneus	**36** Quadratus plantae
27 Talocalcanean part of talocalcaneonavicular joint	**37** Abductor digiti minimi
28 Talonavicular part of talocalcaneonavicular joint	**38** Medial process of tuberosity of calcaneus
29 Cuneonavicular joint	**39** Bursa
30 Cuneometatarsal joint	**40** Tendo calcaneus

Sections of the foot *sagittal sections of the right foot*

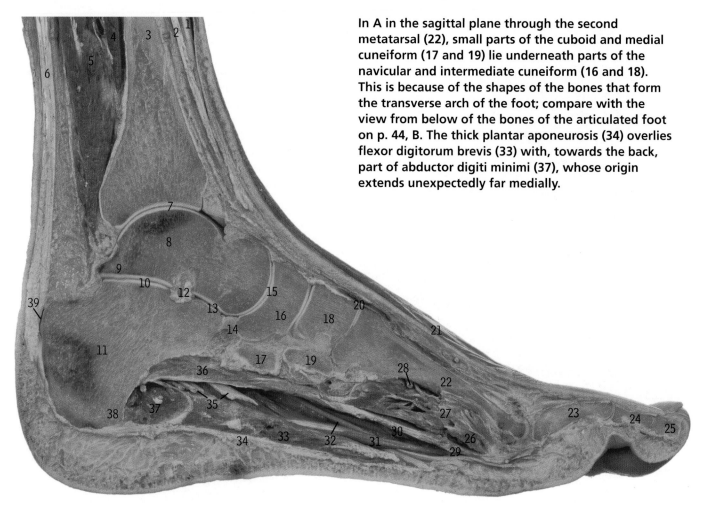

In A in the sagittal plane through the second metatarsal (22), small parts of the cuboid and medial cuneiform (17 and 19) lie underneath parts of the navicular and intermediate cuneiform (16 and 18). This is because of the shapes of the bones that form the transverse arch of the foot; compare with the view from below of the bones of the articulated foot on p. 44, B. The thick plantar aponeurosis (34) overlies flexor digitorum brevis (33) with, towards the back, part of abductor digiti minimi (37), whose origin extends unexpectedly far medially.

A through the second toe, from the lateral side

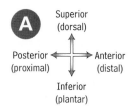

Superior
(dorsal)

A Posterior ◄──────► Anterior
(proximal)   (distal)

Inferior
(plantar)

1	Tibialis anterior	**11**	Calcaneus
2	Extensor hallucis longus	**12**	Interosseous talocalcanean ligament
3	Tibia	**13**	Talocalcanean part of talocalcaneonavicular joint
4	Tibialis posterior	**14**	Plantar calcaneonavicular (spring) ligament
5	Flexor hallucis longus	**15**	Talonavicular part of talocalcaneonavicular joint
6	Tendo calcaneus	**16**	Navicular
7	Ankle joint	**17**	Cuboid
8	Talus	**18**	Intermediate cuneiform
9	Lateral tubercle of talus	**19**	Medial cuneiform
10	Talocalcanean joint	**20**	Extensor digitorum brevis

In B through the sagittal plane of the fifth metatarsal
(47), the tendon of fibularis (*peroneus*) longus (42) is
seen coursing obliquely under the cuboid (17); compare
with 10 on p. 91.

compare
with 10 on p. 91.

21 Extensor digitorum longus tendon to second toe
22 Second metatarsal
23 Proximal
24 Middle ⎱ phalanx of second toe
25 Distal ⎰
26 Transverse head ⎱ of adductor hallucis
27 Oblique head ⎰
28 Plantar arch
29 Second lumbrical overlying flexor digitorum longus tendon to
   second toe
30 Flexor digitorum longus tendon to third toe
31 Flexor digitorum brevis tendon to second toe
32 Second common plantar digital nerve
33 Flexor digitorum brevis
34 Plantar aponeurosis
35 Lateral plantar nerve and vessels
36 Quadratus plantae
37 Abductor digiti minimi
38 Medial process of tuberosity of calcaneus
39 Bursa
40 Lateral branch of superficial fibular (*peroneal*) nerve
41 Fibula
42 Fibularis (*peroneus*) longus
43 Fibularis (*peroneus*) brevis
44 Lateral process of tuberosity of calcaneus
45 Calcaneocuboid joint
46 Cuboideometatarsal joint
47 Fifth metatarsal
48 Flexor digiti minimi brevis
49 Metatarsophalangeal joint of fifth toe

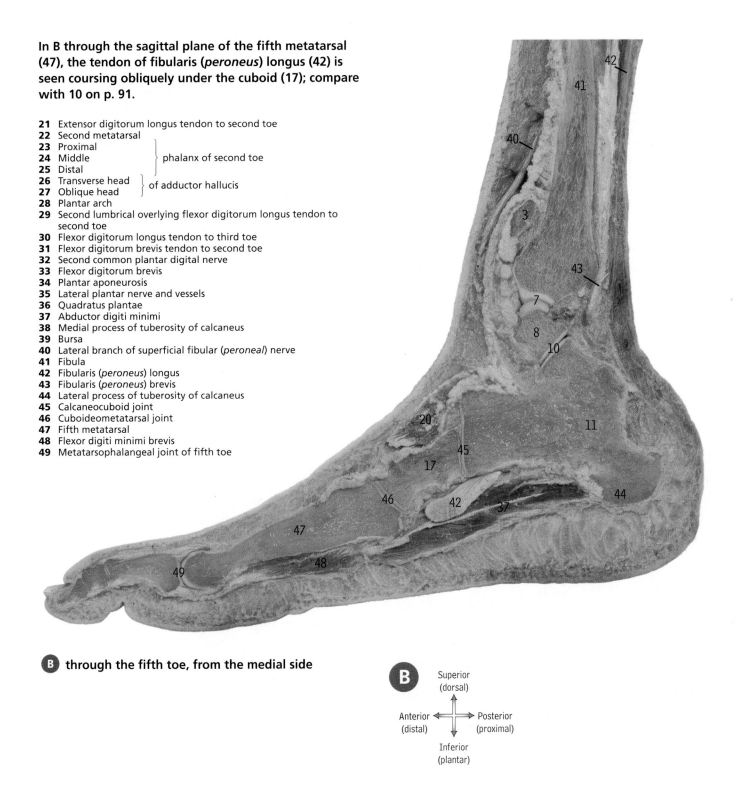

B **through the fifth toe, from the medial side**

B

Superior
(dorsal)

Anterior ⟷ Posterior
(distal)   (proximal)

Inferior
(plantar)

Sections of the foot *sections and images of the right lower leg and foot*

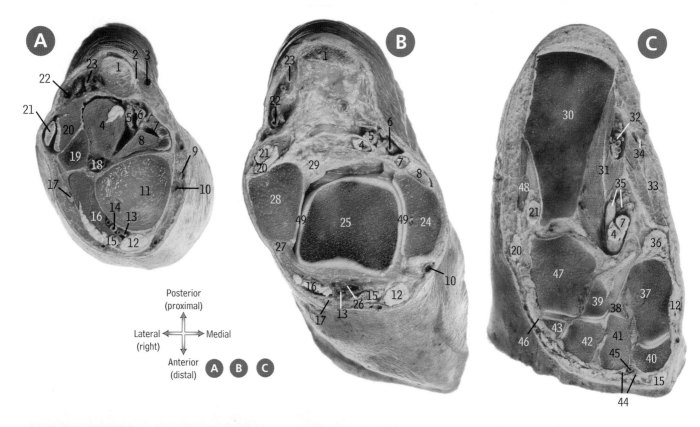

Posterior
(proximal)

Lateral ⟷ Medial
(right)

Anterior
(distal)   A   B   C

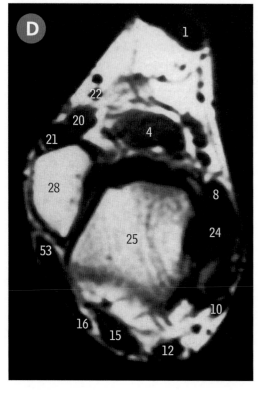

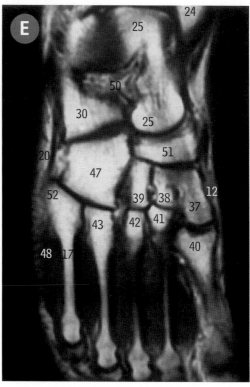

A axial section 6 cm above the ankle joint

B axial section through the ankle joint

C oblique section 5 cm below the ankle joint

D axial magnetic resonance image (MRI) of the ankle joint

E axial magnetic resonance image (MRI) of the foot

Above the ankle in A fibularis (*peroneus*) brevis (20) is behind the fibula (19) with the tendon of fibularis (*peroneus*) longus (21) lying laterally, but at the lower levels in B and C the tendon of fibularis (*peroneus*) longus (21) is behind that of fibularis (*peroneus*) brevis (20). The lowest part of flexor hallucis longus (4) is seen arising from the fibula (19).

At the level of the medial malleolus (24) in B, the tendon of tibialis posterior (8) lies adjacent to the bone, with the tendon of flexor digitorum longus (7) immediately behind it. The posterior tibial vessels (6) and the tibial nerve (5) intervene between the digitorum tendon (7) and the tendon of flexor hallucis longus (4). At the front of the medial malleolus (24) in B, note the great saphenous vein (10), and in front of the talus (25) the dorsalis pedis artery (26) and deep fibular (*peroneal*)

nerve (13) lie between the tendons of extensor hallucis longus (15) and extensor digitorum longus (16).

In the oblique section in C the cuboid (47) lies in front of the calcaneus (30), and at a lower level the tendon of fibularis (*peroneus*) longus (21) will pass underneath the cuboid. On the medial side behind the medial cuneiform (37) the very tip of the tuberosity of the navicular (36) receives the main attachment of tibialis posterior. The tendons of flexor hallucis longus (4) and flexor digitorum longus (7) are more laterally placed.

The sections A, B and C are viewed from above, looking from the knee towards the ankle.

Compare the MRI in D with the section in B, and E with C; the images are at similar but not identical levels.

1   Tendo calcaneus
2   Plantaris
3   A tributary of great saphenous vein
4   Flexor hallucis longus
5   Tibial nerve
6   Posterior tibial vessels
7   Flexor digitorum longus
8   Tibialis posterior
9   Saphenous nerve
10 Great saphenous vein
11 Tibia
12 Tibialis anterior
13 Deep fibular (*peroneal*) nerve
14 Anterior tibial vessels
15 Extensor hallucis longus
16 Extensor digitorum longus
17 Superficial fibular (*peroneal*) nerve
18 Fibular (*peroneal*) vessels
19 Fibula
20 Fibularis (*peroneus*) brevis
21 Fibularis (*peroneus*) longus
22 Small saphenous vein
23 Sural nerve
24 Medial malleolus
25 Talus
26 Dorsalis pedis artery
27 Anterior talofibular ligament

28 Lateral malleolus
29 Posterior talofibular ligament
30 Calcaneus
31 Quadratus plantae
32 Lateral plantar nerve and vessels
33 Abductor hallucis
34 Medial calcanean nerve
35 Medial plantar nerve and vessels
36 Tip of tuberosity of navicular and tibialis posterior
37 Medial   ⎫
38 Intermediate ⎬ cuneiform
39 Lateral   ⎭
40 First   ⎫
41 Second   ⎬ metatarsal base
42 Third   ⎮
43 Fourth   ⎭
44 First dorsal interosseus
45 Deep plantar artery
46 Extensor digitorum brevis
47 Cuboid
48 Abductor digiti minimi
49 Ankle joint
50 Tarsal sinus
51 Navicular
52 Tuberosity of base of fifth metatarsal
53 Fibularis (*peroneus*) tertius

Sections of the foot
Coronal sections of the left ankle joint and foot (in plantarflexion)

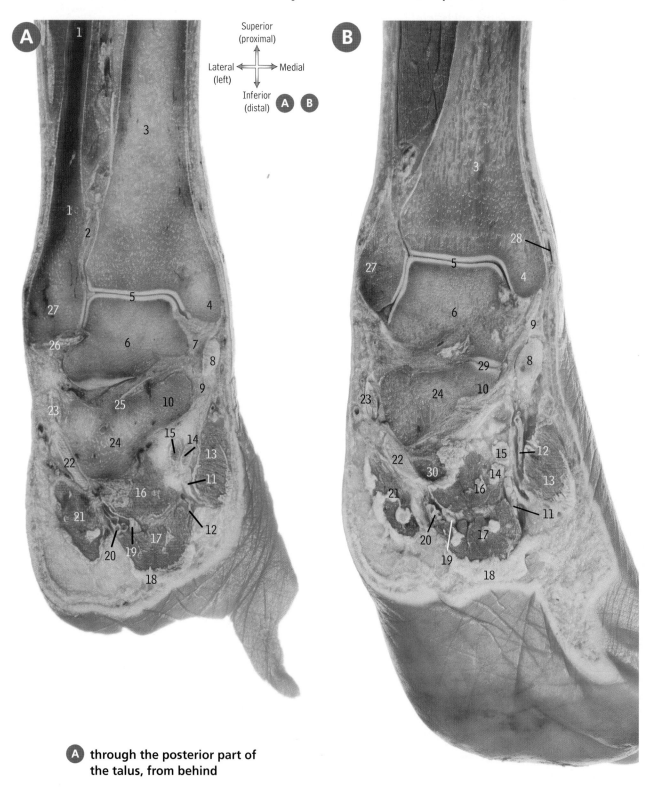

A   through the posterior part of
the talus, from behind

B   about 1 cm in front of A, through the talocalcanean
part of the talocalcaneonavicular joint, from behind

These coronal sections through the ankle joint (5) emphasize how the talus (6) is gripped between the two malleoli (27 and 4). In A the interosseous talocalcanean ligament (25) lies between the talus (6) and calcaneus (24), while in B the section has passed through the part of the sustentaculum tali (10), which forms the talocalcanean part of the talocalcaneonavicular joint (29). In the center of the sole in both sections flexor digitorum brevis (17) overlies quadratus plantae (16); the fusion of plantae with the tendon of flexor digitorum longus (14) is shown in B, where the tendon of flexor hallucis longus (15) has come to lie deep to the digitorum tendon (compare with the dissection B on p. 85 and the section B on p. 102).

- **Joints, muscles and movements:**
  At the ankle joint

  Dorsiflexion: tibialis anterior, extensor hallucis longus, extensor digitorum longus, fibularis (*peroneus*) tertius.
  Plantarflexion: gastrocnemius, soleus, plantaris, tibialis posterior, flexor hallucis longus, flexor digitorum longus.

  At the talocalcanean and talocalcaneonavicular joints

  Inversion: tibialis anterior and tibialis posterior.
  Eversion: fibularis (*peroneus*) longus, fibularis (*peroneus*) brevis and fibularis (*peroneus*) tertius.

- At the other small joints of the foot there are minor degrees of gliding or rotatory movements. At the transverse tarsal joint (p. 51) a small amount of inversion and eversion occurs, but by far the greater part of these important movements takes place at the two joints beneath the talus. To visualize inversion and eversion, imagine the talus held firmly between the tibia and fibula, and the whole of the rest of the foot swivelling inwards or outwards underneath the talus. These movements do not take place at the ankle joint, which essentially only allows dorsiflexion and plantarflexion.

- The actions of muscles on the toes are indicated by their names but the part played by the interossei and lumbricals requires some explanation (apart from the abduction and adduction produced by the interossei and referred to on p. 87). Briefly the interossei and lumbricals work together to flex the metatarsophalangeal joints and extend the interphalangeal joints; these apparently contradictory actions on different joints by the same muscles can be explained as follows.

- The interossei (both plantar and dorsal) are attached mainly to the sides of the proximal phalanges but also into the dorsal digital expansions; the lumbricals are usually attached entirely to the expansions. Because of the position of these attachments in relation to the axis of movement of the metatarsophalangeal joints, the interossei and lumbricals plantarflex these joints.

- Because the lumbrical attachments and parts of the interosseus attachments are to the basal angles of the expansions, the line of pull is transmitted to the dorsal surfaces of the toes distal to the metatarsophalangeal joints, and so the interphalangeal joints are extended.

- In most feet the interosseus attachment to the expansion is minimal, and it is the lumbricals that are mainly responsible for assisting the long and short extensor tendons in extending the toes, keeping them straight and stabilized against the pull of the flexors, which tend to make them buckle, especially during the push-off phase of walking when flexor hallucis longus and flexor digitorum longus are contracting strongly.

1 Fibula
2 Interosseous tibiofibular ligament
3 Tibia
4 Medial malleolus
5 Ankle joint
6 Talus
7 Deep part of medial (deltoid) ligament
8 Tibialis posterior
9 Medial ligament
10 Sustentaculum tali
11 Medial plantar nerve
12 Medial plantar artery
13 Abductor hallucis
14 Flexor digitorum longus
15 Flexor hallucis longus
16 Quadratus plantae
17 Flexor digitorum brevis
18 Plantar aponeurosis
19 Lateral plantar nerve
20 Lateral plantar vessels
21 Abductor digiti minimi
22 Fibularis (*peroneus*) longus
23 Fibularis (*peroneus*) brevis
24 Calcaneus
25 Interosseous talocalcanean ligament
26 Posterior talofibular ligament
27 Lateral malleolus
28 Great saphenous vein
29 Talocalcanean part of talocalcaneonavicular joint
30 Cuboid

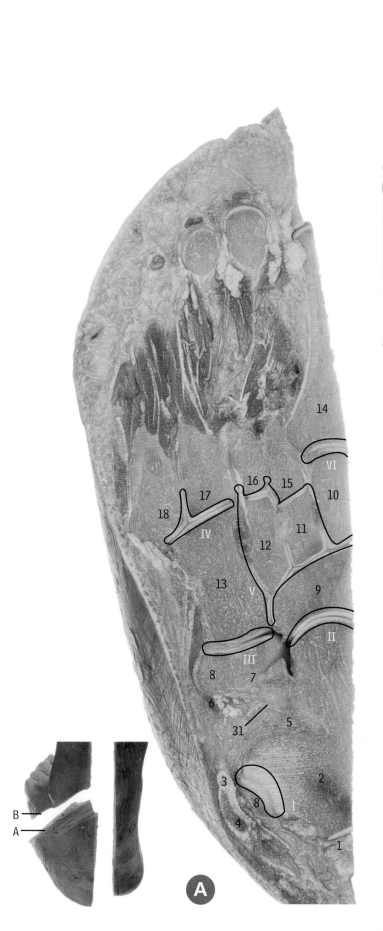

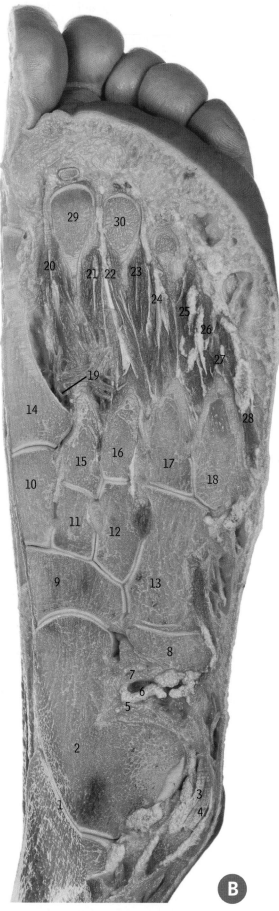

Sections of the foot *oblique axial sections of the left foot*

The plane of section is shown in the small illustration. The surfaces A and B have been separated and are viewed like two pages in an open book.

Between the tarsal bones in A the various joint cavities, outlined in black and numbered with Roman figures, are explained in the notes below.

In B the navicular (9) is seen between the talus (2) and the three cuneiforms (10–12). Note how the base of the second metatarsal (15) projects more proximally than the bases of the first and third metatarsals (14 and 16). On the lateral side the cuboid (13) articulates at the back with the very small part of the calcaneus (8) seen in this section, and at the front with the bases of the fourth and fifth metatarsals (17 and 18). Parts of all the interosseus muscles (four dorsal and three plantar, 20–26) are identified in the forefoot.

1 Ankle joint
2 Talus
3 Fibularis (*peroneus*) brevis
4 Fibularis (*peroneus*) longus
5 Interosseous talocalcanean ligament
6 Extensor digitorum brevis
7 Cervical ligament
8 Calcaneus
9 Navicular
10 Medial ⎫
11 Intermediate ⎬ cuneiform
12 Lateral ⎭
13 Cuboid
14 First ⎫
15 Second ⎪
16 Third ⎬ metatarsal base
17 Fourth ⎪
18 Fifth ⎭
19 Deep plantar branch of first dorsal metatarsal artery
20 First dorsal ⎫
21 Second dorsal ⎪
22 First plantar ⎪
23 Third dorsal ⎬ interosseus
24 Second plantar ⎪
25 Fourth dorsal ⎪
26 Third plantar ⎭
27 Flexor digiti minimi brevis
28 Abductor digiti minimi
29 Head of second metatarsal
30 Head of third metatarsal
31 Inferior extensor retinaculum

- The cavities of a number of synovial joints in the foot are continuous with one another to the extent that there are normally six synovial cavities associated with the tarsal bones:

  I   The talocalcanean joint cavity.
  II   The talocalcaneonavicular joint cavity.
  III   The calcaneocuboid joint cavity.
  IV   The cuboideometatarsal joint cavity (between the cuboid and the bases of the fourth and fifth metatarsals).
  V   The cuneonavicular and cuneometatarsal joint cavity (between the navicular, the three cuneiforms and the bases of the second, third and fourth metatarsals).
  VI   The medial cuneometatarsal joint cavity (between the medial cuneiform and the base of the first metatarsal).

- Parts of all the above cavities can be seen in the foot sectioned here; they are indicated by the black lines in **A** and numbered as above. (The cuboideonavicular joint is usually a fibrous union but in this specimen it is synovial and continuous with the cuneonavicular joint cavity.)

Sections of the foot *coronal sections of the tarsus of the right foot*

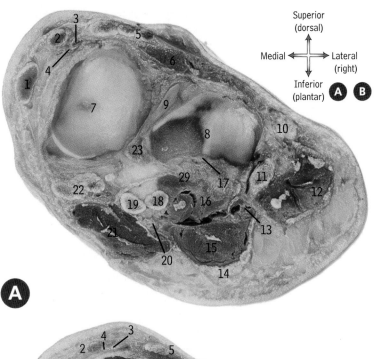

Superior
(dorsal)

Medial ←——→ Lateral
(right)

Inferior
(plantar)   Ⓐ Ⓑ

Ⓐ

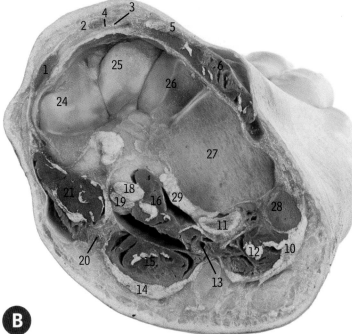

Ⓑ

Ⓐ through the transverse tarsal joint, proximal to the navicular

Ⓑ through the cuneonavicular joint, distal to the navicular

Both sections are viewed from behind, looking from the heel toward the toes.

In A the section has passed through the talonavicular joint, so displaying the posterior (proximal) surface of the navicular (7). A small part of the cuboid (8) has been sliced off, leaving cartilage on the more lateral part of its posterior (calcanean) surface. The plantar aponeurosis (14) overlies flexor digitorum brevis (15), with abductor hallucis (21) on the medial side and abductor digiti minimi (12) laterally. Quadratus plantae (16) lies centrally, with the tendons of flexor hallucis longus (18) and flexor digitorum longus (19) more medially placed at this level.

In B at the level of the posterior (navicular) surfaces of the cuneiform bones, the tendon of flexor hallucis longus (18) is now passing deep to the digitorum tendon (19). The tendon of fibularis (*peroneus*) longus (11) is turning laterally under the cuboid (27), where a little more distally it will become covered by the long plantar ligament (29) (compare with the dissection on p. 91).

1 Tibialis anterior
2 Extensor hallucis longus
3 Dorsalis pedis artery
4 Deep fibular (*peroneal*) nerve
5 Extensor digitorum longus
6 Extensor digitorum brevis
7 Posterior articular surface of navicular (for talus)
8 Posterior articular surface of cuboid (for calcaneus)
9 Anterior tip of calcaneus
10 Fibularis (*peroneus*) brevis
11 Fibularis (*peroneus*) longus
12 Abductor digiti minimi
13 Lateral plantar nerve and vessels
14 Plantar aponeurosis
15 Flexor digitorum brevis
16 Quadratus plantae
17 Plantar calcaneocuboid (short plantar) ligament
18 Flexor hallucis longus
19 Flexor digitorum longus
20 Medial plantar nerve and vessels
21 Abductor hallucis
22 Tibialis posterior
23 Plantar calcaneonavicular (spring) ligament
24 Medial ⎫
25 Intermediate ⎬ cuneiform
26 Lateral ⎭
27 Cuboid
28 Tuberosity of fifth metatarsal
29 Long plantar ligament

coronal sections of the right metatarsus

Both sections are viewed from behind, looking toward the toes. The metatarsals are numbered in Roman figures. On the dorsum the tendons of extensor digitorum longus to the appropriate toes are numbered L2–L5, and those of extensor digitorum brevis B2–B4 (recall that the brevis tendon to the great toe is named extensor hallucis brevis, 2). Similarly in the sole the flexor digitorum longus tendons are numbered L2–L5,

with the lumbrical muscles that arise from those tendons numbered U1–U4. The various interosseus muscles between and below the metatarsals have not been labeled.

In B note the sesamoid bones (18) under the head of the first metatarsal (I), with the tendon of flexor hallucis longus (8) between them.

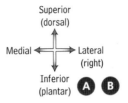

Superior
(dorsal)

Medial ◄─────► Lateral
(right)

Inferior
(plantar)　Ⓐ Ⓑ

1 Extensor hallucis longus
2 Extensor hallucis brevis
3 Arcuate artery
4 Deep plantar artery
5 Abductor hallucis
6 Proper plantar digital nerve of great toe
7 Flexor hallucis brevis
8 Flexor hallucis longus
9 Oblique head of adductor hallucis
10 Second plantar metatarsal artery
11 Flexor digiti minimi brevis
12 Abductor digiti minimi
13 Common plantar digital branches of medial plantar nerve
14 Plantar aponeurosis
15 Deep branch of lateral plantar nerve
16 Fourth common plantar digital nerve
17 Proper plantar digital nerve of fifth toe
18 Sesamoid bone
19 Transverse head of adductor hallucis

Ⓐ **through the middle of the metatarsal shafts**

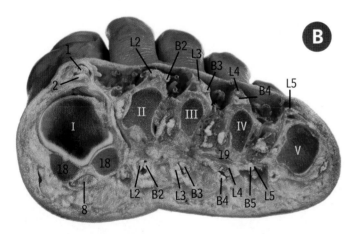

Ⓑ **through the heads of the first and fifth metatarsals**

Great toe
The dorsum, nail, and sections of the great toe

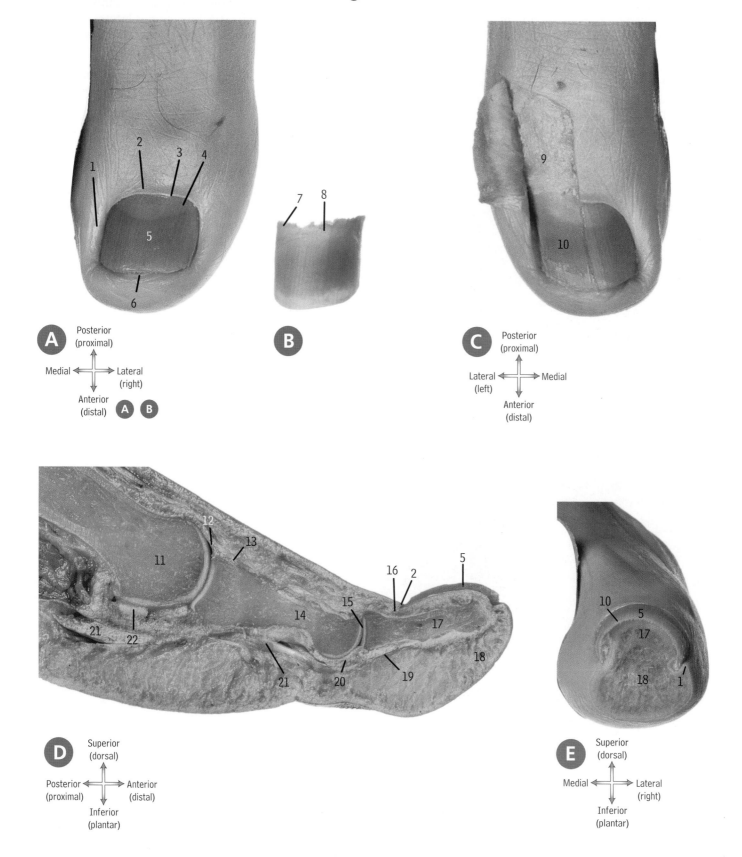

A
Posterior
(proximal)

Medial ⟷ Lateral
(right)

Anterior
(distal) **A** **B**

B

C
Posterior
(proximal)

Lateral ⟷ Medial
(left)

Anterior
(distal)

D
Superior
(dorsal)

Posterior ⟷ Anterior
(proximal)   (distal)

Inferior
(plantar)

E
Superior
(dorsal)

Medial ⟷ Lateral
(right)

Inferior
(plantar)

A dorsum of the right great toe

B nail

C nail bed of the left great toe

D sagittal section of the right great toe, from the lateral side

E coronal section of the distal phalanx of the right great toe

1 Nail wall
2 Nail fold
3 Eponychium
4 Lunule ⎫
5 Body ⎪
6 Free border ⎬ of nail
7 Occult border ⎪
8 Root ⎭
9 Germinal matrix ⎫ of nail bed
10 Sterile matrix ⎭
11 Head of first metatarsal
12 Capsule of metatarsophalangeal joint
13 Attachment of extensor hallucis brevis
14 Proximal phalanx
15 Capsule of interphalangeal joint
16 Attachment of extensor hallucis longus
17 Distal phalanx
18 Septa of pulp space
19 Attachment of flexor hallucis longus
20 Plantar ligament of interphalangeal joint
21 Flexor hallucis longus
22 Sesamoid bone

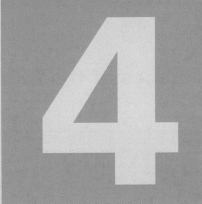

Imaging of the Foot and Ankle

Images of the foot and ankle

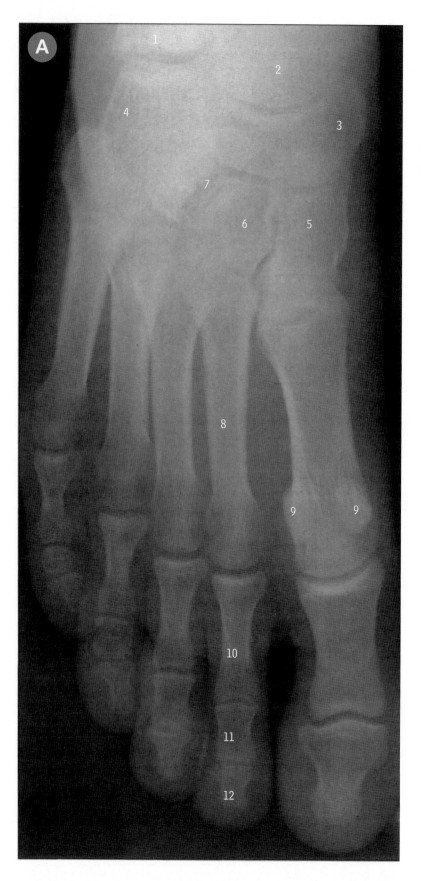

Radiographs

A from above (dorsoplantar view)

B lateral view

The view in A looks down on to the dorsum of the right foot in front of the ankle, while the side view in B shows the ankle and other adjacent joints.

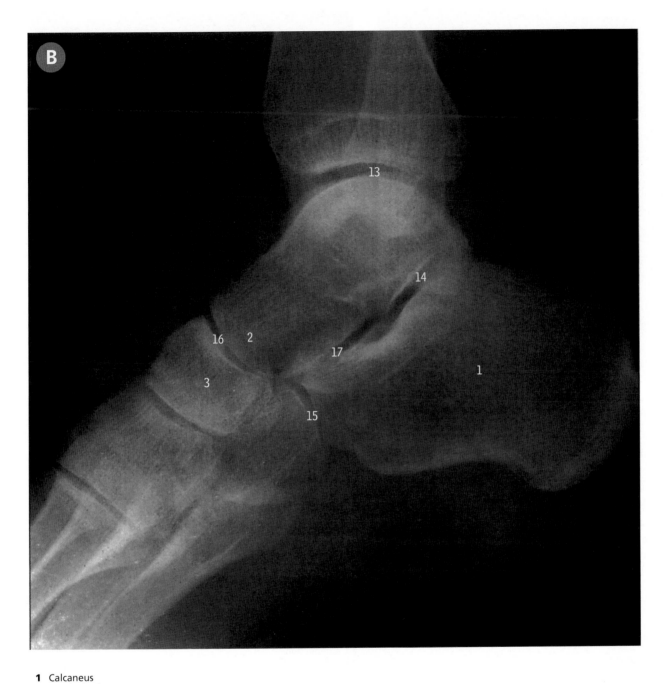

1 Calcaneus
2 Head of talus
3 Navicular
4 Cuboid
5 Medial ⎫
6 Intermediate ⎬ cuneiform
7 Lateral ⎭
8 Second metatarsal
9 Sesamoid bone
10 Proximal ⎫
11 Middle ⎬ phalanx of second toe
12 Distal ⎭
13 Ankle joint
14 Talocalcaneal joint (posterior facet)
15 Calcaneocuboid joint
16 Talonavicular part ⎫
17 Talocalcanean part ⎬ of talocalcaneonavicular joint

Images of the foot and ankle *ankle and foot joints*

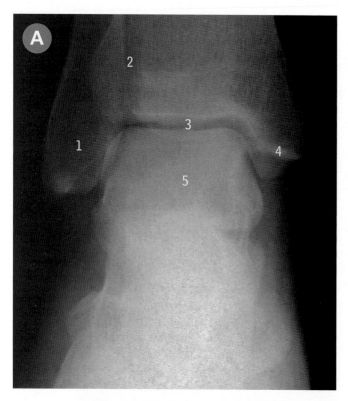

A   anteroposterior radiograph

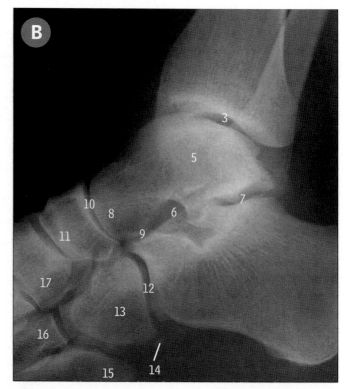

B   lateral radiograph

In A the talus (5) is embraced by the lateral and medial malleoli (1 and 4) and the lower end of the tibia, giving a very evenly-spaced ankle joint line (3).

The lateral view in B shows the tarsal sinus (6) between the talus and calcaneus, with the talocalcaneal joint (7) behind the sinus and the talocalcanean part (9) of the talocalcaneonavicular joint in front of it. The talonavicular part of the talocalcaneonavicular joint is in

front of the head of the talus (8). Behind the cuboid (13) is the calcaneocuboid joint (12), and in front of it the articulations with the fourth and fifth metatarsals (15 and 16). Below the cuboid is a small (occasional) sesamoid bone in the tendon of fibularis (*peroneus*) longus (14).

Compare the metatarsals and sesamoid bones in C and D with those on p. 44.

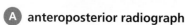

1	Lateral malleolus
2	Inferior tibiofibular joint
3	Ankle joint
4	Medial malleolus
5	Talus
6	Tarsal sinus
7	Talocalcaneal joint (posterior facet)
8	Head of talus
9	Talocalcanean part } of talocalcaneonavicular joint
10	Talonavicular part

11	Navicular bone
12	Calcaneocuboid joint
13	Cuboid bone
14	Sesamoid bone in tendon of fibularis (*peroneus*) longus
15	Tuberosity of base of fifth metatarsal
16	Base of fourth metatarsal
17	Cuneiform bones

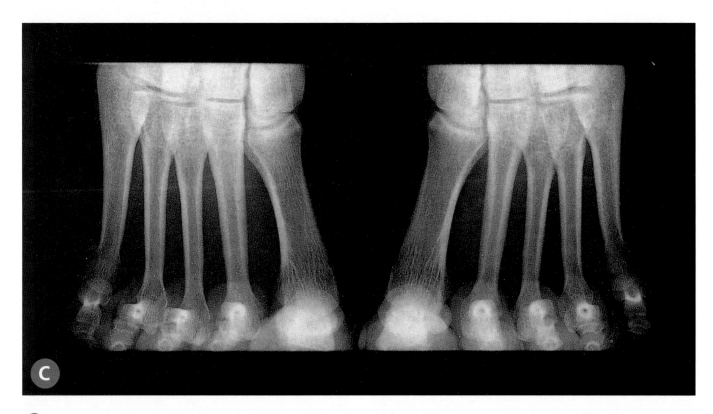

C radiograph standing on tip-toe

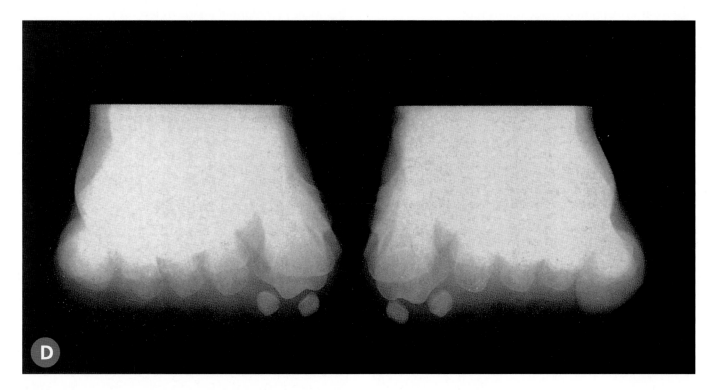

D radiograph to show sesamoid bones under great toes

Magnetic Resonance Images (MRIs) *Axial (transverse) sections through the left foot*

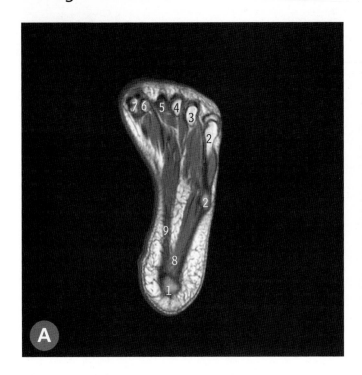

A axial T1-weighted image of left foot

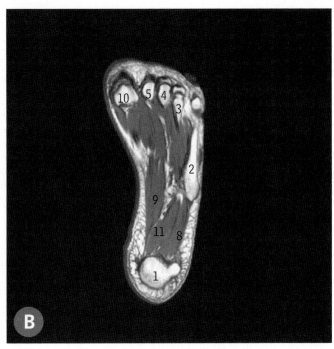

B axial T1-weighted image of left foot

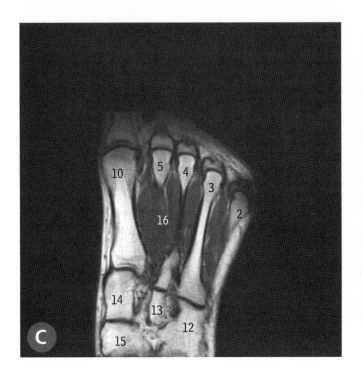

C axial T1-weighted image of left foot

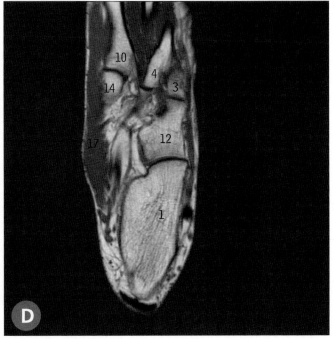

D axial T1-weighted image of left foot

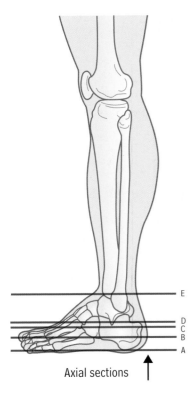

Axial sections

1 Calcaneus
2 Fifth ⎫
3 Fourth ⎬ metatarsal
4 Third ⎪
5 Second ⎭
6 Lateral sesamoid bone
7 Medial sesamoid bone (bipartite)
8 Abductor digiti minimi
9 Flexor digitorum brevis
10 First metatarsal
11 Quadratus plantae
12 Cuboid
13 Lateral ⎫ cuneiform
14 Medial ⎬
15 Navicular
16 Interosseus muscles
17 Abductor hallucis
18 Medial malleolus of tibia
19 Talus
20 Lateral malleolus of fibula
21 Tibialis anterior
22 Extensor hallucis longus
23 Extensor digitorum longus
24 Fibularis (peroneus) brevis
25 Fibularis (peroneus) longus
26 Flexor hallucis longus
27 Tendo calcaneus (Achilles' tendon)
28 Tibialis posterior
29 Flexor digitorum longus

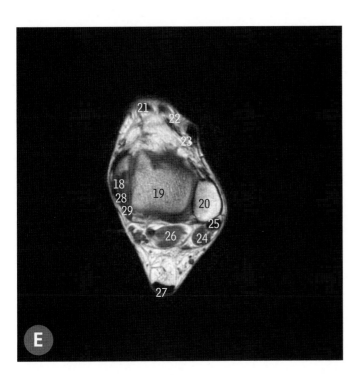

E axial T1-weighted image of left foot

Magnetic Resonance Images (MRIs) *sagittal sections through the left foot*

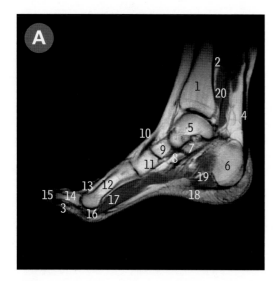

A sagittal T1-weighted image of left foot

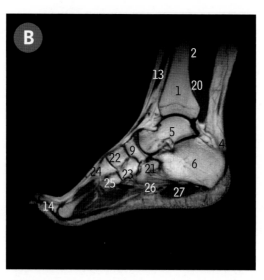

B sagittal T1-weighted image of left foot

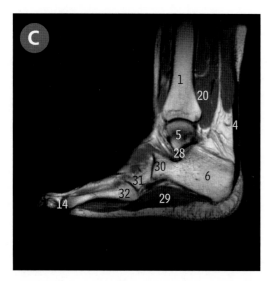

C sagittal T1-weighted image of left foot

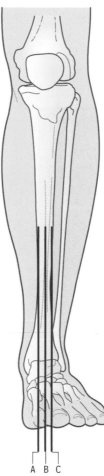

Sagittal sections

1 Tibia
2 Tibialis posterior
3 Flexor digitorum longus
4 Tendo calcaneus (Achilles' tendon)
5 Talus
6 Body ⎫
7 Sustenaculum tali ⎬ of calcaneus
8 Spring ligament
9 Navicular
10 Tibialis anterior
11 Medial cuneiform
12 First metatarsal
13 Extensor hallucis longus
14 Proximal phalanx
15 Distal phalanx
16 Sesamoid bone
17 Flexor hallucis brevis
18 Plantar aponeurosis
19 Abductor hallucis
20 Flexor hallucis longus
21 Cuboid
22 Intermediate ⎫
23 Lateral ⎬ cuneiform
24 Second ⎫
25 Third ⎬ metatarsal
26 Short plantar ligament
27 Quadratus plantae
28 Posterior facet of talocalcaneal joint
29 Abductor digiti minimi
30 Anterior process of calcaneus
31 Cuboid
32 Fifth metatarsal

Magnetic Resonance Images (MRIs) *coronal sections through the left foot*

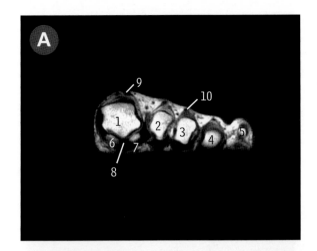

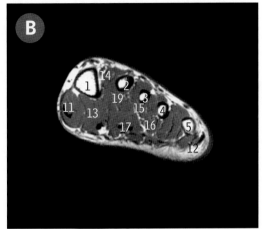

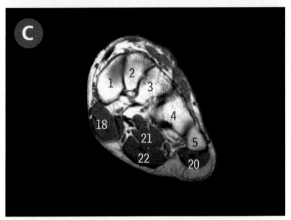

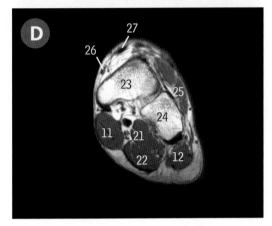

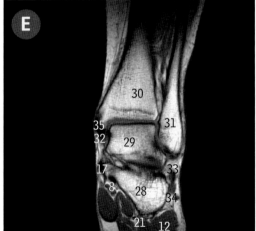

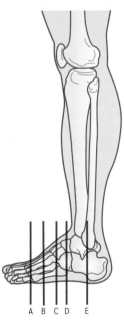

Ⓐ coronal T1-weighted image of left foot

Ⓑ coronal T1-weighted image of left foot

Ⓒ coronal T1-weighted image of left foot

Ⓓ coronal T1-weighted image of left foot

Ⓔ coronal T1-weighted image of left foot

Coronal sections

1 First ⎫
2 Second ⎪
3 Third ⎬ metatarsal
4 Fourth ⎪
5 Fifth ⎭
6 Medial ⎫ sesamoid bone
7 Lateral ⎭
8 Flexor hallucis longus
9 Extensor hallucis longus
10 Extensor digitorum longus to third toe
11 Abductor hallucis
12 Abductor digiti minimi
13 Adductor hallucis
14 First dorsal ⎫
15 First plantar ⎬ interosseus
16 Third plantar ⎭
17 Flexor digitorum longus
18 Flexor hallucis brevis
19 Adductor hallucis (oblique head)
20 Flexor digiti minimi brevis
21 Quadratus plantae
22 Flexor digitorum brevis
23 Talus (neck)
24 Cuboid
25 Extensor digitorum brevis
26 Tibialis anterior
27 Extensor hallucis longus
28 Calcaneus (body)
29 Talus (body)
30 Tibia
31 Fibula
32 Deltoid ligament
33 Fibularis (peroneus) brevis
34 Fibularis (peroneus) longus
35 Tibialis posterior

Appendix

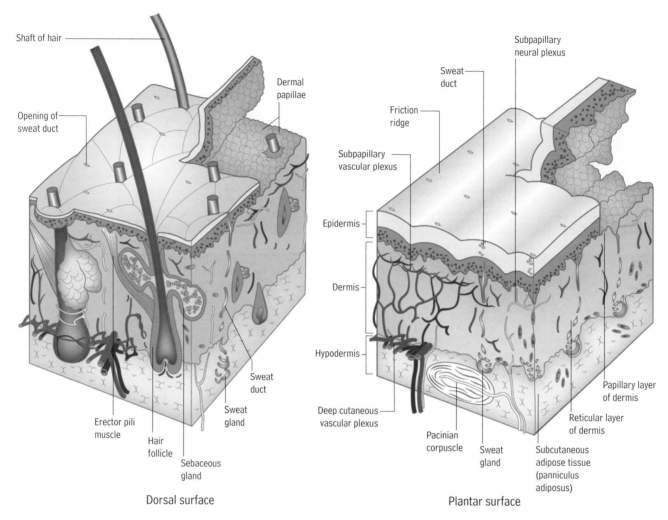

Shaft of hair

Opening of sweat duct

Dermal papillae

Erector pili muscle

Hair follicle

Sebaceous gland

Sweat gland

Sweat duct

Dorsal surface

Sweat duct

Friction ridge

Subpapillary vascular plexus

Epidermis

Dermis

Hypodermis

Deep cutaneous vascular plexus

Pacinian corpuscle

Sweat gland

Subpapillary neural plexus

Papillary layer of dermis

Reticular layer of dermis

Subcutaneous adipose tissue (panniculus adiposus)

Plantar surface

Fig. 1 Schematic diagram comparing the structures present in the thin and hairy dorsal skin and those in the thick, hairless plantar skin of the foot. The epidermis has been partially reflected to show epidermal and dermal papillae.

SKIN

The skin of the dorsal and plantar surfaces of the foot differ in appearance and organization (see Fig 1).

MUSCLES

MUSCLES OF THE GLUTEAL REGION

Gluteus maximus

From the posterior gluteal line of the hip bone, the dorsal surface of the lower part of the sacrum and the side of the coccyx, the sacrotuberous ligament, and the fascia over gluteus medius

To the iliotibial tract, with the deep fibres of the lower part attaching to the gluteal tuberosity of the femur

Inferior gluteal nerve, L5, S1, 2

Extension and lateral rotation of the hip joint

Gluteus medius

From the outer surface of the ilium between the posterior and anterior oblique lines

To the lateral surface of the greater trochanter of the femur

Superior gluteal nerve, L4, 5, S1

Abduction and medial rotation of the hip joint, and prevention of adduction

Gluteus minimus

From the outer surface of the ilium between the anterior and inferior gluteal lines

To the anterior part of the lateral surface of the greater trochanter of the femur

Superior gluteal nerve, L4, 5, S1

Abduction and medial rotation of the hip joint, and prevention of adduction

Piriformis
From the middle three pieces of the sacrum
To the upper border of the greater trochanter of the
femur
Branches from L5, S1, 2
Abduction, lateral rotation and stabilization of the hip
joint

Quadratus femoris
From the upper part of the outer border of the ischial
tuberosity
To the quadrate tubercle of the intertrochanteric crest of
the femur
Nerve to quadratus femoris, L4, 5, S1
Lateral rotation and stabilization of the hip joint

Obturator internus
From the inner surface of the obturator membrane and
the adjacent anterolateral pelvic wall
To the greater trochanter of the femur, above and in
front of the trochanteric fossa
Nerve to obturator internus, L5, S1, 2
Lateral rotation and stabilization of the hip joint

Gemellus superior and inferior
Superior from the dorsal surface of the ischial spine,
inferior from the upper part of the ischial tuberosity
To the superior and inferior borders respectively of
obturator internus
Nerves to obturator internus (superior) and quadratus
femoris (inferior)
Assists obturator internus

Obturator externus
From the outer surface of the obturator membrane and
the ischiopubic ramus
To the trochanteric fossa of the femur
Obturator nerve, L3, 4,
Lateral rotator of the thigh

MUSCLES OF THE FRONT OF THE THIGH

Iliacus
From the upper two-thirds of the iliac fossa in the lower
abdomen
To the psoas tendon and the femur below and in front of
the lesser trochanter
Femoral nerve, L2, 3
Flexor of the hip, assisting psoas major

Psoas major
From the sides of the lumbar vertebrae and intervertebral
discs
To the lesser trochanter of the femur
Branches from L1, 2, 3
Flexor of the hip

Tensor fasciae latae
From the anterior 5 cm of the outer lip of the iliac crest
To the iliotibial tract
Superior gluteal nerve, L4, 5, S1
Extensor of the knee and lateral rotator of the leg

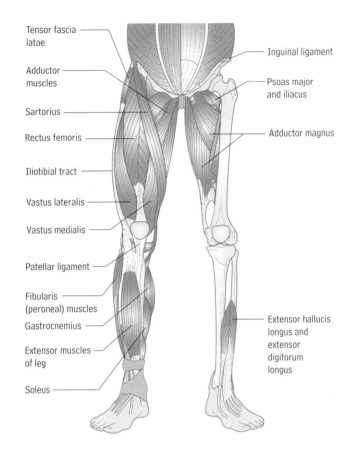

Fig. 2 Muscles: From the front. Superficial muscles on the right side of
the body; deep muscles on the left side.

Sartorius
From the anterior superior iliac spine
To the upper part of the medial surface of the shaft of
the tibia in front of gracilis and semitendinosus
Femoral nerve, L2, 3
Flexor, adductor and lateral rotator of the hip

Rectus femoris
From the anterior inferior iliac spine (straight head) and the
ilium above the rim of the acetabulum (reflected head)
To the base of the patella
Femoral nerve, L3, 4
Flexor of the hip and extensor of the knee

Vastus lateralis
From the upper part of the intertrochanteric line of the
femur, anterior and inferior borders of the greater
trochanter, lateral lip of the gluteal tuberosity and the
upper part of the linea aspera
To the lateral border of the patella and the quadriceps
tendon
Femoral nerve, L2, 3, 4
Extensor of the knee

Vastus medialis

From the lower part of the intertrochanteric line of the
femur, the spiral line, the linea aspera, the upper part
of the medial supracondylar line and the tendon of
adductor magnus
To the medial border of the patella and the quadriceps
tendon
Femoral nerve, L2, 3, 4
Extensor of the knee

Vastus intermedius

From the anterior and lateral surfaces of the upper two-
thirds of the shaft of the femur
To the deep part of the quadriceps tendon
Femoral nerve, L2, 3, 4
Extensor of the knee

Articularis genus

From the anterior surface of the femur below vastus
intermedius
To the apex of the suprapatellar bursa
Femoral nerve, L3, 4
Retraction of the bursa as the knee extends

MUSCLES OF THE MEDIAL SIDE OF THE THIGH

Pectineus

From the pectineal line of the pubis and bone in front of
the line
To the femur on a line from the lesser trochanter to the
linea aspera
Femoral nerve, L2, 3
Flexor, adductor and lateral rotator of the hip

Gracilis

From the body of the pubis and ischiopubic ramus
To the upper part of the medial surface of the shaft of
the tibia, between sartorius and semitendinosus
Obturator nerve, L2, 3
Flexor, adductor and medial rotator of the thigh

Adductor brevis

From the body and inferior ramus of the pubis
To the shaft of the femur on a line from the lesser
trochanter to the linea aspera, and to the upper part of
the linea
Obturator nerve, L2, 3, 4
Adductor of the thigh

Adductor longus

From the front of the pubis
To the middle part of the linea aspera
Obturator nerve, L2, 3, 4
Adductor of the thigh

Adductor magnus

From the lower lateral part of the ischial tuberosity and
the ischiopubic ramus
To the shaft of the femur from the gluteal tuberosity
along the linea aspera to the medial supracondylar line,
and to the adductor tubercle
Obturator nerve, L2, 3, 4 and sciatic nerve, L4, 5, S1
Adductor and lateral rotator of the thigh

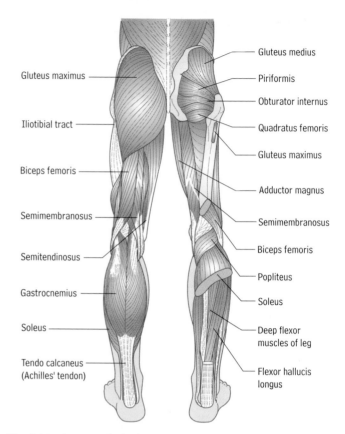

Fig. 3 Muscles: From the back. Superficial muscles on the left side of the
body; deep muscles on the right side.

MUSCLES OF THE BACK OF THE THIGH

Biceps femoris

From the medial facet of the ischial tuberosity with
semimembranosus (long head) and from the linea
aspera and lateral supracondylar line of the femur
(short head)
To the head of the fibula
Sciatic nerve (*tibial* part to long head, common fibular
(*peroneal*) part to short head), L5, S1
Flexion and lateral rotation of the knee and extension of
the hip

Semitendinosus

From the medial facet of the ischial tuberosity, with the
long head of biceps
To the upper part of the subcutaneous surface of the
tibia, behind gracilis
Sciatic nerve (*tibial* part), L5, S1
Flexion and medial rotation of the knee, and extension of
the hip

Semimembranosus

From the lateral facet of the ischial tuberosity
To the groove on the back of the medial condyle of the
tibia, with expansions forming the oblique popliteal
ligament and the fascia over popliteus
Sciatic nerve (*tibial* part), L5, S1
Flexion and medial rotation of the knee, and extension of
the hip

MUSCLES OF THE FRONT OF THE LEG

Tibialis anterior
From the upper two-thirds of the lateral surface of the tibia and adjoining part of the interosseus membrane
To the medial surfaces of the medial cuneiform and base of the first metatarsal
Deep fibular (peroneal) nerve, L4, 5
Dorsiflexion and inversion of the foot

Extensor hallucis longus
From the middle third of the medial surface of the fibula
To the base of the distal phalanx of the great toe
Deep fibular (peroneal) nerve, L4, 5
Extension of the great toe and dorsiflexion of the foot

Extensor digitorum longus
From the upper two-thirds of the medial surface of the fibula
To the four lateral toes by the dorsal digital expansions, attached to the middle and distal phalanges
Deep fibular (peroneal) nerve, L5, S1
Extension of the second to fifth toes and dorsiflexion of the foot

Fibularis (*peroneus*) tertius
From the lower third of the medial surface of the fibula, continuous with extensor digitorum longus
To the shaft of the fifth metatarsal
Deep fibular (peroneal) nerve, L5, S1
Dorsiflexion and eversion of the foot

MUSCLE OF THE DORSUM OF THE FOOT

Extensor digitorum brevis
From the upper surface of the calcaneus
To the base of the proximal phalanx of the great toe (as extensor hallucis brevis) and the dorsal digital expansions of the second to fourth toes
Deep fibular (peroneal) nerve, L5, S1
Extension of the first to fourth toes

MUSCLES OF THE LATERAL SIDE OF THE LEG

Fibularis (*peroneus*) longus
From the upper two-thirds of the lateral surface of the fibula
To the lateral sides of the medial cuneiform and base of the first metatarsal
Superficial fibular (peroneal) nerve, L5, S1, 2
Plantarflexion and eversion of the foot

Fibularis (*peroneus*) brevis
From the lower two-thirds of the lateral surface of the fibula
To the tuberosity of the base of the fifth metatarsal
Superficial fibular (peroneal) nerve, L5, S1, 2
Plantarflexion and eversion of the foot

MUSCLES OF THE BACK OF THE LEG

Gastrocnemius
Medial head from the upper posterior part of the medial condyle of the femur; lateral head from the lateral surface of the lateral condyle of the femur
To the middle of the posterior surface of the calcaneus by the tendo calcaneus (in association with soleus)
Tibial nerve, S1, 2
Plantarflexion of the foot and flexion of the knee

Soleus
From the soleal line and upper part of the medial border of the tibia, a tendinous arch over the popliteal vessels and tibial nerve, and the upper part of the posterior surface of the fibula
To the tendo calcaneus with gastrocnemius (see above)
Tibial nerve, S1, 2
Plantarflexion of the foot

Plantaris
From the lateral supracondylar line of the femur
To the calcaneus on the medial side of the tendo calcaneus
Tibial nerve, S1, 2
Plantarflexion of the foot and weak flexion of the knee

Popliteus
From the back of the tibia above the soleal line
To the outer surface of the lateral epicondyle of the femur
Tibial nerve, L4, 5, S1
Lateral rotation of the femur on the fixed tibia (or medial rotation of the tibia on the fixed femur); pulls lateral meniscus backward during flexion of the knee

Tibialis posterior
From the posterior surface of the interosseous membrane and adjacent posterior surfaces of the tibia and fibula
To the tuberosity of the navicular, with slips to other tarsal bones (except the talus) and the middle three metatarsals
Tibial nerve, L4, 5
Plantarflexion and inversion of the foot

Flexor hallucis longus
From the lower two-thirds of the posterior surface of the fibula
To the plantar surface of the base of the distal phalanx of the great toe
Tibial nerve, S2, 3
Plantarflexion of the great toe and foot

Flexor digitorum longus
From the medial part of the posterior surface of the tibia below the soleal line
To the four lateral toes by a tendon to each, reaching the plantar surface of the base of the distal phalanx
Tibial nerve, S2, 3
Plantarflexion of the four lateral toes and foot

MUSCLES OF THE SOLE OF THE FOOT

FIRST LAYER

Abductor hallucis
From the medial process of the calcanean tuberosity and the plantar aponeurosis
To the medial side of the proximal phalanx of the great toe
Medial plantar nerve, S2, 3
Abduction and plantarflexion of the great toe

Flexor digitorum brevis
From the medial process of the calcanean tuberosity and the deep surface of the central part of the plantar aponeurosis
To the lateral four toes by a tendon to each; the tendon divides into two slips (to allow the flexor digitorum longus tendon to pass between them), which are attached to the sides of the middle phalanx
Medial plantar nerve, S2, 3
Plantarflexion of the four lateral toes

Abductor digiti minimi
From the lateral and medial processes of the calcanean tuberosity and the plantar aponeurosis
To the lateral side of the base of the proximal phalanx of the fifth toe (with flexor digiti minimi brevis)
Lateral plantar nerve, S2, 3
Abduction and plantarflexion of the fifth toe

SECOND LAYER

Quadratus plantae
From the (concave) medial surface of the calcaneus and from the plantar surface of the calcaneus in front of the lateral process of the tuberosity
To the lateral border of flexor digitorum longus before the division into four tendons
Lateral plantar nerve, S2, 3
Assistance with plantarflexion of the four lateral toes

Lumbricals
First lumbrical from the medial border of the first tendon of flexor digitorum longus
Second, third and fourth lumbricals from the four adjoining tendons of flexor digitorum longus
To the medial sides of the dorsal digital expansions of the tendons of extensor digitorum longus
First lumbrical—medial plantar nerve; second, third and fourth lumbricals by the lateral plantar nerve, S2, 3
Plantarflexion at the four lateral metatarsophalangeal joints and extension at interphalangeal joints
Tendons of flexor digitorum longus and flexor hallucis longus

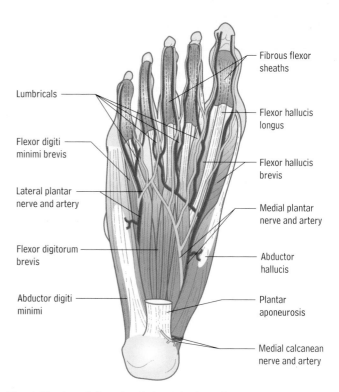

Fig. 4 Muscles of the sole of the right foot: first layer. For dissection see p. 84.

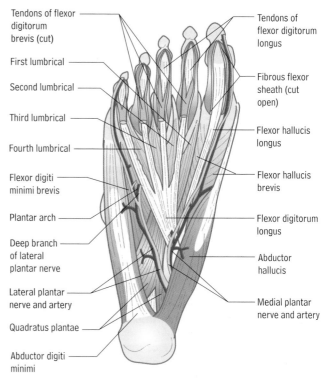

Fig. 5 Muscles of the sole of the right foot: second layer. For dissection see p. 85.

THIRD LAYER

Flexor hallucis brevis

From the plantar surface of the cuboid and lateral cuneiform

By a tendon to each side of the base of the proximal phalanx of the great toe, the medial tendon joining with that of abductor hallucis and the lateral with adductor hallucis; there is a sesamoid bone in each tendon

Medial plantar nerve, S2, 3

Plantarflexion of the metatarsophalangeal joint of the great toe

Adductor hallucis

Oblique head from the bases of the second, third and fourth metatarsals

Transverse head from the plantar metatarsophalangeal ligaments of the third, fourth and fifth toes

To the lateral side of the base of the proximal phalanx of the great toe, with part of flexor hallucis brevis

Lateral plantar nerve, S2, 3

Adduction of the great toe

Flexor digiti minimi brevis

From the plantar surface of the base of the fifth metatarsal

To the lateral side of the base of proximal phalanx of the fifth toe, with abductor digiti minimi

Lateral plantar nerve, S2, 3

Plantarflexion of the metatarsophalangeal joint of the fifth toe

FOURTH LAYER

Dorsal interosseus (four)

From adjacent sides of the bodies of the metatarsals

To the bases of proximal phalanges and the dorsal digital expansions. First and second to the medial and lateral sides of the second toe; third and fourth to the lateral sides of the third and fourth toes

Lateral plantar nerve, S2, 3

Plantarflexion of the metatarsophalangeal joints and extension (dorsiflexion) of the interphalangeal joints of the second, third and fourth toes; abduction of the same toes

Plantar interosseus (three)

From the bases and medial sides of the third, fourth and fifth metatarsals

To the medial sides of the bases of the proximal phalanges and dorsal digital expansions of the corresponding toes

Lateral plantar nerve, S2, 3

Plantarflexion of the metatarsophalangeal joints and extension (dorsiflexion) of the interphalangeal joints of the third, fourth and fifth toes; adduction of the same toes

Tendons of tibialis posterior and fibularis (*peroneus*) longus

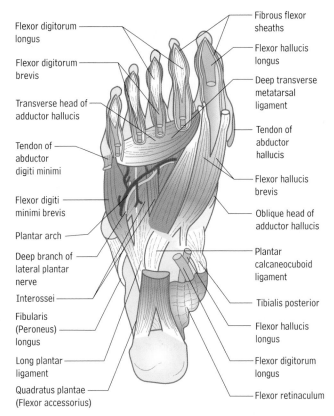

Fig. 6 Muscles of the sole of the right foot: third layer. For dissection see p. 86.

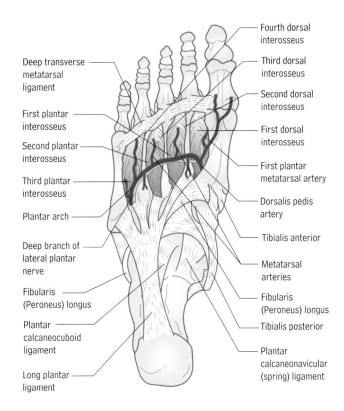

Fig. 7 Muscles of the sole of the right foot: fourth layer. For dissection see p. 87.

NERVES

BRANCHES OF THE LUMBAR PLEXUS

Muscular T12, L1, 2, 3, 4 to psoas major and minor, quadratus lumborum and iliacus

Iliohypogastric and ilio-inguinal L1 to parts of internal oblique and transversus abdominis in anterior abdominal wall

Genitofemoral L1, 2, giving off
Genital branch (to cremaster muscle of spermatic cord)
Femoral branch

Lateral cutaneous of thigh L2, 3

Femoral L2, 3, 4, giving off
Nerve to pectineus
Anterior division, giving off
Intermediate femoral cutaneous
Medial femoral cutaneous
Nerve to sartorius
Posterior division, giving off
Saphenous
Nerves to quadriceps femoris

Obturator L2, 3, 4, giving off
Anterior branch
Muscular to adductor longus, adductor brevis and gracilis
Posterior branch
Muscular to obturator externus and adductor magnus
Accessory obturator (occasional) L3, 4 to pectineus

BRANCHES OF THE SACRAL PLEXUS

Superior gluteal L4, 5, S1, to gluteus medius, gluteus minimus and tensor fasciae latae

Inferior gluteal L5, S1, 2, to gluteus maximus

Nerve to piriformis S1, 2

Nerve to quadratus femoris and gemellus inferior L4, 5, S1

Nerve to obturator internus and gemellus superior L5, S1, 2

Posterior femoral cutaneous S2, 3

Sciatic nerve L4, 5, S1, 2, 3 giving off
Muscular branches to biceps, semimembranosus, semitendinosus and part of adductor magnus
Tibial nerve—see below
Common fibular (*peroneal*) nerve—see below

Perforating cutaneous, pudendal and other pelvic and perineal branches

BRANCHES OF THE TIBIAL NERVE L4, 5, S1, 2, 3

Muscular to gastrocnemius, plantaris, soleus, popliteus, tibialis posterior, flexor digitorum longus and flexor hallucis longus

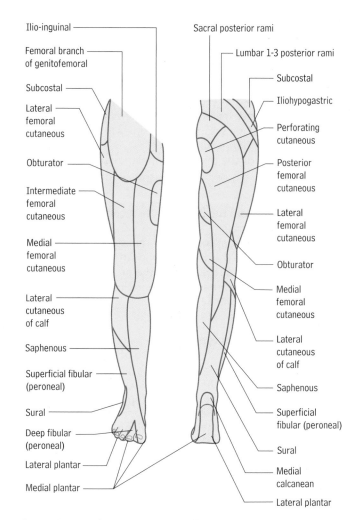

Fig. 8 Diagram of cutaneous nerves of the front and back of the right lower limb.

Sural (ending as lateral dorsal cutaneous and then dorsal digital to lateral side of fifth toe)
Medial calcanean
Medial plantar—see below
Lateral plantar—see below

BRANCHES OF THE COMMON FIBULAR (*PERONEAL*) NERVE L4, 5, S1, 2

Recurrent
Lateral cutaneous of calf
Fibular (peroneal) communicating

Superficial fibular (peroneal), giving off
  Muscular to fibularis (*peroneus*) longus and fibularis
  (*peroneus*) brevis
  Medial branch (medial dorsal cutaneous), giving off
    Dorsal digital
  Lateral branch (intermediate dorsal cutaneous),
  giving off
    Dorsal digital
Deep fibular (peroneal), giving off
  Muscular to tibialis anterior, extensor hallucis longus,
  extensor digitorum longus and fibularis (*peroneus*)
  tertius
  Lateral terminal, to extensor digitorum brevis
  Medial terminal, giving off
    Dorsal digital (to first cleft)

BRANCHES OF THE MEDIAL PLANTAR NERVE L4, 5, S1

Trunk giving off
  Nerve to abductor hallucis
  Nerve to flexor digitorum brevis
Proper plantar digital nerve of great toe, giving off
  Nerve to flexor hallucis brevis.
First common plantar digital nerve, giving off
  Nerve to first lumbrical
  Proper plantar digital nerves of first cleft
Second common plantar digital nerve, giving off
  Proper plantar digital nerves of second cleft
Third common plantar digital nerve, giving off
  Proper plantar digital nerves of third cleft

BRANCHES OF THE LATERAL PLANTAR NERVE S1, 2

Trunk, giving off
  Nerve to quadratus plantae
  Nerve to abductor digiti minimi
Superficial branch, giving off
  Fourth common plantar digital nerve, giving off
    Proper plantar digital nerves of fourth cleft
  Proper plantar digital nerve of fifth toe, giving off
    Nerve to flexor digiti minimi brevis
    Nerve to third plantar interosseus
    Nerve to fourth dorsal interosseus
Deep branch, giving off
  Nerve to adductor hallucis
  Nerves to second, third and fourth lumbricals
  Nerves to first, second and third dorsal interossei
  Nerves to first and second plantar interossei

REGIONAL ANAESTHESIA OF THE FOOT

For operations on the front part of the foot, one or more
of the five nerves that supply the foot—tibial, saphenous,

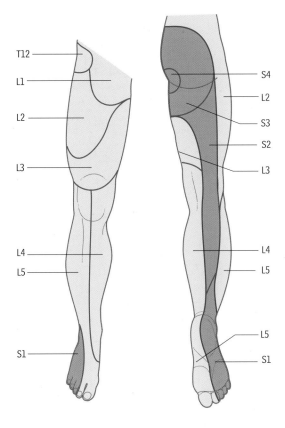

Fig. 9 Diagram of dermatomes of the front and back of the right lower limb. (A dermatome is the area of skin supplied by any one spinal nerve.) Note that both the dorsum and sole of the foot are supplied by L5 and S1 dermatomes.

superficial fibular (*peroneal*), deep fibular (*peroneal*) and sural—can be infiltrated with local anaesthetic. The object is to deliver the solution adjacent to the nerve trunks so that it can diffuse into them from the surrounding tissue; the nerves themselves must not be penetrated by the needle. In all cases before injection of the anaesthetic solution, aspiration must be attempted to ensure that the needle tip has not entered a blood vessel.

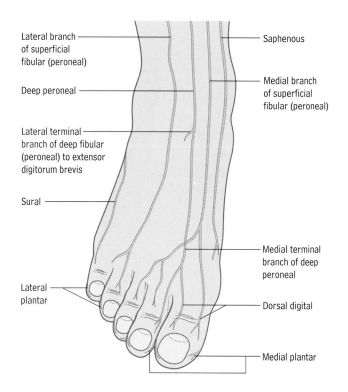

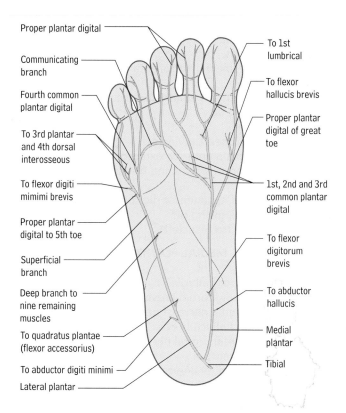

Fig. 10 Diagram of nerves of the dorsum of the right foot. Note that the tips of the toes are supplied from the sole by digital branches of the medial and lateral plantar nerves; their terminations curl round onto the dorsum of the toes in the region of the nails.

Fig. 11 Diagram of branches of the right medial and lateral plantar nerves. The medial plantar nerve gives off branches to four of the muscles of the sole (abductor hallucis, flexor digitorum brevis, flexor hallucis brevis and the first lumbrical); all the other muscles of the sole are supplied by the lateral plantar nerve (see the notes on p. 78). Often, as shown here, there is a communicating branch between the adjacent plantar digital branches of the medial and lateral plantar nerves.

Tibial nerve

For infiltration of the tibial nerve behind the medial malleolus (p. 76), the needle is inserted at the medial edge of the tendo calcaneus (Achilles' tendon), 2 cm above the tip of the medial malleolus and at right angles to the tibia. The needle is advanced until it touches the tibia and is then withdrawn slightly; the object is to allow the solution to percolate into the neurovascular compartment deep to the flexor retinaculum.

Saphenous and superficial fibular (*peroneal*) nerves

The saphenous and superficial fibular (*peroneal*) nerves can be infiltrated as they approach the dorsum of the foot between the two malleoli (p. 68). The needle is inserted in front of the medial malleolus and is directed transversely and subcutaneously toward the lateral malleolus, deep to the superficial veins but superficial to the extensor tendons.

Deep fibular (*peroneal*) nerve

The deep fibular (*peroneal*) nerve can be infiltrated at the level of the middle of the tarsus as it lies between the tendon of extensor hallucis longus and the second toe tendon of extensor digitorum longus (p. 78). The needle is inserted perpendicular to the dorsum, between the tendons and lateral to the dorsalis pedis artery (if present and palpable), so that the solution infiltrates the tissues over the first intermetatarsal space.

Sural nerve

The sural nerve can be infiltrated above and behind the tip of the lateral malleolus by a needle inserted lateral to the tendo calcaneus (Achilles' tendon) and directed perpendicularly toward the fibularis (*peroneus*) longus tendon, avoiding the small saphenous vein (p. 71).

ARTERIES

BRANCHES OF THE FEMORAL ARTERY

Giving off the following before becoming the popliteal
    artery
Superficial epigastric
Superficial circumflex iliac
Superficial external pudendal
Deep external pudendal
Profunda femoris, giving off
    Lateral circumflex femoral
    Medial circumflex femoral
    Perforating
Descending genicular

BRANCHES OF THE POPLITEAL ARTERY

Sural
Superior, middle and inferior genicular
Anterior tibial, giving off the following before becoming
    the dorsalis pedis artery (see below)
    Posterior and anterior tibial recurrent
    Anterior medial and anterior lateral malleolar
Posterior tibial, giving off
    Circumflex fibularis
    Fibular (*peroneal*), giving off
        Nutrient to the fibula
        Perforating
        Communicating
        Lateral malleolar
        Calcanean
    Nutrient to the tibia
    Communicating
    Medial malleolar
    Calcanean
    Medial plantar—see below
    Lateral plantar—see below

BRANCHES OF THE DORSALIS PEDIS ARTERY

Lateral tarsal
Medial tarsal
First dorsal metatarsal, giving off
    Deep plantar (perforating) branch, to complete plantar
      arch
    Dorsal digital branch to medial side of great toe
    Dorsal digital branches of first cleft

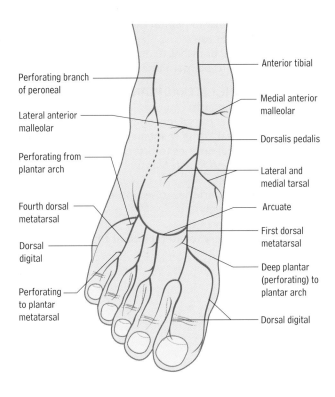

Fig. 12 Diagram of branches of the right dorsalis pedis artery, excluding muscular and most anastomotic branches, but note that anastomoses from the perforating branch of the fibular (*peroneal*) artery may link up with the arcuate artery and enlarge to replace an absent dorsalis pedis artery.

Arcuate, giving off
    Second dorsal metatarsal, giving off
        Perforating branches
        Dorsal digital branches to second cleft
    Third dorsal metatarsal, giving off
        Perforating branches
        Dorsal digital branches to third cleft
    Fourth dorsal metatarsal, giving off
        Perforating branches
        Dorsal digital branches to fourth cleft
        Dorsal digital branch to lateral side of fifth toe

BRANCHES OF THE MEDIAL PLANTAR ARTERY

Anastomotic branch to plantar digital artery of medial
    side of the great toe
Superficial digital branches to anastomose with first,
    second and third plantar metatarsal arteries

BRANCHES OF THE LATERAL PLANTAR ARTERY

Plantar arch, giving off
    First plantar metatarsal, giving off
        Plantar digital artery to medial side of great toe
        Plantar digital arteries to first cleft
    Second, third and fourth plantar metatarsal arteries,
        each giving off
        Plantar digital arteries to second, third and fourth
        clefts respectively
    Perforating branches
Plantar digital artery to lateral side of fifth toe

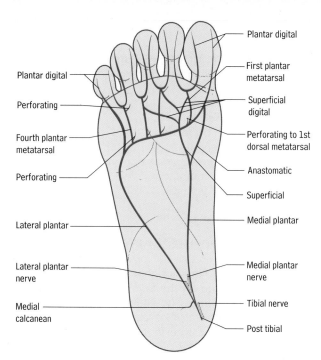

Fig. 13 Diagram of branches of the right medial and lateral plantar arteries (excluding muscular and most anastomotic branches). The proximal parts of the medial and lateral plantar nerves are shown in green to indicate that the nerves lie on the internal sides of their corresponding arteries.

Index